CREATIVE
ENGAGEMENT
IN OCCUPATION

Building Professional Skills

CREATIVE
ENGAGEMENT
IN OCCUPATION

Building Professional Skills

Authors

Margaret S. Coffey, MA, COTA, ROH
Academic Fieldwork Coordinator/ Instructor
Occupational Therapy Assistant Program
Brown Mackie College-South Bend
South Bend, Indiana

Nancy K. Lamport, MS, OTR
Associate Professor Emeritus
Department of Occupational Therapy
School of Health and Rehabilitation Sciences
Indianapolis, Indiana

Gayle I. Hersch, PhD, OTR
Professor, School of Occupational Therapy
Texas Woman's University
Houston, Texas

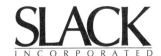

www.Healio.com/books

ISBN: 978-1-61711-039-9

Creative Engagement in Occupation includes ancillary materials specifically available for faculty use. Included are PowerPoint slides. Please visit www.efacultylounge.com to obtain access.

SLACK Incorporated uses a review process to evaluate submitted material. Prior to publication, educators or clinicians provide important feedback on the content that we publish. We welcome feedback on this work.

Published by: SLACK Incorporated
                  6900 Grove Road
                  Thorofare, NJ 08086 USA
                  Telephone: 856-848-1000
                  Fax: 856-848-6091
                  www.Healio.com/books

Contact SLACK Incorporated for more information about other books in this field or about the availability of our books from distributors outside the United States.

Library of Congress Cataloging-in-Publication Data

Creative engagement in occupation : building professional skills / [edited by] Margaret S. Coffey, Nancy K. Lamport, Gayle I. Hersch.
    p. ; cm.
Includes bibliographical references and index.
ISBN 978-1-61711-039-9 (alk. paper)
I. Coffey, Margaret S., - , editor. II. Lamport, Nancy K., - , editor. III. Hersch, Gayle Ilene, editor.
[DNLM: 1. Occupational Therapy--methods. 2. Creativity. 3. Professional Practice. WB 555]
RM735
615.8'515--dc23
                        2014043553

Printed in the United States of America.

Last digit is print number: 10 9 8 7 6 5 4 3 2 1

DEDICATION

In honor of those who believed and fostered growth in our creative abilities, this book is dedicated to Donald Lamport, Arnold Hersch, and Phillip Coffey.

Contents

Creative Engagement in Occupation includes ancillary materials specifically available for faculty use. Included are PowerPoint slides. Please visit www.efacultylounge.com to obtain access.

ACKNOWLEDGMENTS

We gratefully acknowledge the guidance and support of Brien Cummings, our acquisitions editor, and the staff at SLACK Incorporated, who have provided us the opportunity to create a companion text to *Activity Analysis: Application to Occupation* as a second step in providing professional education. Through their belief in this project, especially during times of excessive professional and personal demands, we were able to realize our vision for this book. We are also indebted to the expertise and research of our invited colleagues at Texas Woman's University (Dallas and Houston), whose writing on the use of creativity in occupational therapy greatly contributed to the value and scope of this text: Mary Frances Baxter, PhD, LOT, FAOTA, Harriett A. Davidson, MA, OTR, Tina Fletcher, EdD, MFA, OTR, and Marsha Neville, PhD, MS, OT.

We extend our appreciation to the students of the Master's Program of Occupational Therapy at Texas Woman's University and the Associate Degree Occupational Therapy Assistant Program of Brown Mackie College (South Bend, IN) for their help in the development and refinement of discussion questions, exercises, activities, assignments, and examples of completed work. Special praise goes to Michelle S. Scheffler, MOT, for providing a current chart of the *OTPF* components and literature review. We thank Cissette Muster, MOT, for her valuable help in completing many secretarial tasks. We are also grateful to students Marisa Barra, Kate Campbell, Lauri Chupp, Kembe Frederick, Stephanie Mareska, Cindia Reyes, Alisha Romero, Kelly Smith, Kate Swope, and Alex Tesmer for permission to use samples of their completed assignments. In addition, we would like thank our TWU students, Laura Homan, MOTS and Emily Stevens, MOTS, for their assistance with edits.

Finally, we gratefully express our love and appreciation to the very special people in our lives who have provided steady encouragement while we wrestled with the demands of time and energy to bring this project to publication.

ABOUT THE AUTHORS

Margaret S. Coffey, MA, COTA, ROH is the Academic Fieldwork Coordinator and a Faculty Instructor in the Occupational Therapy Assistant Program at Brown Mackie College (South Bend, IN). She received her BA degree in biology at Wheaton College, her AS degree in occupational therapy technology at Indiana University School of Health and Rehabilitation Sciences (formerly known as the Occupational Therapy Program, School of Allied Health Sciences, Indiana University School of Medicine, Indianapolis), and her MA degree in art at the University of Indianapolis. Her specialty areas of practice are in psychiatric hospital settings, long-term care, and residential facilities for adults experiencing dementia. Her teaching responsibilities are in the areas of therapeutic media, group activities, mental health, and geriatrics. She serves as a consultant and facilitator for experiences in the adult population at Moon Tree Studios, an outreach ministry exploring the interconnectedness of art, nature, and spirituality in Donaldson, IN.

Nancy K. Lamport, MS, OTR is Associate Professor Emeritus in the Department of Occupational Therapy School of Health and Rehabilitation Sciences (Indianapolis, IN) (formerly known as the Occupational Therapy Program, School of Allied Health Sciences, Indiana University School of Medicine, Indianapolis). She received her BS degree in occupational therapy at Ohio State University and her MS degree in special education at Butler University (Indianapolis, IN). She was a preschool teacher for 7 years in Indianapolis and worked as an occupational therapist at the Commission for Handicapped Children in Kentucky and the Veteran's Hospital in Louisville, KY. Prior to her retirement, her teaching responsibilities included the fundamentals of occupational therapy (activity analysis), activities of daily living skills, leisure activities, and media. Together with her husband, she established the Horizon Fund to provide funding for the professional development of occupational therapy students to attend the American Occupational Therapy Association National Student Conclaves and IOTA State conferences.

Gayle I. Hersch, PhD, OTR is Professor with the School of Occupational Therapy at Texas Woman's University (Houston, TX). She received her BS degree in occupational therapy, her MS degree in allied health sciences, and her PhD in educational psychology at Indiana University. Her practice area is in gerontology with an emphasis on Alzheimer's disease, stroke, caregiving, and home safety. Her current responsibilities are in the areas of teaching and research with MOT and PhD students. Her content emphasis is on geriatric practice, qualitative methodology, and adaptation to relocation to residential settings. Efforts to tap into student creativity have been done in coursework via experiential activities and with the development of research grants and client intervention protocols.

Contributing Authors

Mary Frances Baxter, PhD, LOT, FAOTA (Chapter 4) is Associate Professor at Texas Woman's University. She received her BS in occupational therapy from Colorado State University, her MA in rehabilitation technology from Texas Woman's University, and her PhD in kinesiology and health from the University of Houston. Her research and practice background and interests include pediatrics, adult neurological patients, oncology, and assistive technology. She infuses creativity in all areas of practice. She currently teaches neuroscience at the entry level and the PhD level for occupational therapy students. In addition, she has taught and given presentations on the neuroscience of occupation, adaptation, and creativity.

Harriett A. Davidson, MA, OTR (Chapter 5) is Associate Professor with the School of Occupational Therapy at Texas Woman's University with responsibilities in the areas of teaching and research. Her more than 50 years of practice as an occupational therapist have included a variety of settings and populations, and she has taught at the associate's and graduate levels, with an emphasis on mental health. She has offered courses in creativity in research and in occupational therapy practice. Her other research has addressed adaptation to relocation and the role of hope in therapy.

Tina Fletcher, EdD, MFA, OTR (Chapter 7, Appendix C) is Assistant Professor in the School of Occupational Therapy at the Texas Woman's University T. Boone Pickens Institute of Health Sciences. Her research interests include creativity and the impact of art media on well-being. She holds a doctoral degree in curriculum design and a master's degree in figurative sculpture and is certified in the administration and interpretation of the Torrance Test of Creative Thinking.

Marsha Neville, PhD, MS, OT (Chapter 3) is Associate Professor in the School of Occupational Therapy at Texas Woman's University. She earned her BS in occupational therapy from Eastern Michigan University, an MS in applied cognition and neuroscience, and a PhD in cognition and neuroscience from the University of Texas at Dallas. Her knowledge of cognitive functioning in everyday occupations has led to a research focus on translational research related to cognitive and physical rehabilitation across the continuum of care for stroke survivors. She has more than 35 years of clinical experience in adult rehabilitation with a focus on persons with acquired brain injuries. She uses creative problem solving in her own practice and challenges her students with exercises that enhance their awareness of thinking creatively.

PREFACE

The motivation for writing this book grew out of our desire to further expand the process begun in *Activity Analysis: Application to Occupation* (2005). Its purpose was to serve as an introduction to the clinical reasoning process for designing occupational therapeutic intervention. The first text provided the student with a method for understanding and applying activity analysis to occupational therapy practice. This second text fosters and engages the student in developing the creative component of the clinical reasoning process to develop a creative approach to intervention. We identify and emphasize the use of creativity as an intrinsic element of occupational therapy education. While both texts stand alone, they complement each other in providing opportunities for students to build professional skills within the framework of occupational therapy practice.

As evident in our historical roots, creative action and problem solving are significant elements in the clinical reasoning process for delivering occupational therapy services. Occupational therapy practitioners originate collaborative relationships with clients to approach and achieve outcomes in diverse ways, as identified in the *Occupational Therapy Practice Framework (OTPF), 2nd Edition* (American Occupational Therapy Association, 2008). Throughout the occupational therapy process, practitioners provide service to clients through a creative synthesis of activity analysis of the client's occupational performance while supporting health and life participation through each of the *OTPF* domain components. The conscious use of the practitioner's own creativity and enlistment of the client as a partner in the therapy process are the keys for successful intervention. Therese Schmid (2005), Doris Pierce (2001), and Estelle Breines (2004) have documented the importance of creativity in delivering occupational therapy services in multiple arenas. The purpose of this text is to help students recognize, enhance, and use their own creativity in the practice of occupational therapy. By including concepts of creativity in preparatory coursework, the student's potential for creative treatment intervention is identified individually, expanded upon through peer participation, and incorporated into case study treatment applications.

The creative process is a significant factor in providing effective treatment for the client and empowering the adult client's own problem-solving skills. Understanding activities through analysis as presented in the authors' first text, *Activity Analysis: Application to Occupation, 5th Edition* (2005), is the beginning of this process. Encouraging the student's ability to think creatively as the client strives to engage in meaningful occupation is the next step. Throughout this text, the student will recognize, explore, and experience the use of creativity in building entry-level performance in this aspect of clinical reasoning. Students assess aspects of their own creative capacities and cognitive components involved in the creative process. Didactic and experiential exercises, discussion questions, and specific assignments are included by occupational therapy specialists with knowledge and experience in using creative intervention in clinical practice. Examples of students' projects designed through use of their own creativity are provided. Applications in case studies illustrate the creativity of both the client and the therapist working together to improve functional performance. Four appendices include diagrams for the *OTPF*; a literature review of articles on creativity; a table of quantitative assessment methods in creativity, personality, and work/vocational aspects; and a list of additional resources used in preparation for writing this text.

Level of Content

The level of content of this text can be graded to accommodate associate, master's, and entry-level clinical doctorate degree students.

REFERENCES

American Occupational Therapy Association. (2008). Occupational therapy practice framework: Domain & process (2nd ed.). *American Journal of Occupational Therapy, 62*(6), 625-683.

Breines, E. B. (2004). *Occupational therapy: Activities for practice and teaching.* Philadelphia, PA: Whurr Publishing.

Hersch, G. I., Lamport, N. K., & Coffey, M. S. (2005). *Activity analysis: Application to occupation* (5th ed.). Thorofare, NJ: SLACK Incorporated.

Pierce, D. (2001). Occupation by design: Dimensions, therapeutic power, and creative process. *American Journal of Occupational Therapy, 55*(3), 249-259.

Schmid, T. (2005). *Promoting health through creativity: For professional in health, arts and education.* London, UK: Whurr Publishers.

INTRODUCTION

In *Activity Analysis and Application: Building Blocks of Treatment* (1996), we provided a philosophy for the importance of activity analysis and methods for using purposeful activity as the medium of occupational therapy intervention. We also developed a strategy for connecting purposeful activity with the client experiencing performance skill deficits in a therapeutic application. This functional relationship between the client and the activity depended upon the context and environment in which the client participated.

In this companion text, we lead students through a process of discovering and enlisting their creative potential in using activities to engage their clients in meaningful occupation. The text is designed to be used in a sequential manner, with each chapter introducing ideas and information that link with those in the previous chapters, to help students recognize the role of creativity in delivering occupational therapy interventions. Classroom components are included in the text for students to recognize how creativity influences their everyday lives and to provide opportunities to become creative in their academic learning, performing activities with others, and realizing their educational goals. Individual and peer exercises, discussions, and problem-solving assignments are provided in each chapter to reveal the students' own creativity. An understanding of the role of creativity in the history of occupational therapy, the cognitive and neurological components of creativity, and current research in creativity provides a foundation for the clinical reasoning process. Student examples of using creativity to complete projects are included as further inspiration for using one's potential to be creative.

Creativity is an important attribute in clinical reasoning skills. The creative process is routinely used by practitioners for choosing a treatment approach to mirror clients' needs, for providing "just-right" challenges to motivate clients to participate, and for identifying how clients will succeed in their present or future context and environment. Experiential activities in the text provide a baseline to which students can compare their personal growth as occupational therapy practitioners. For example, when the instructor role plays symptoms of a stroke to a student, it can simulate working with a client with similar deficits. The student can perform an activity normally and then examine performance of the same activity with the change in the client's ability as a result of the medical condition. A client with left-sided weakness who needs to perform a task in which bilateral coordination is required, who has poor recall of multistep instructions given orally, or who has impaired vision that leads to an illegible signature offers opportunities to create alternative approaches. Experiencing the physical differences in performance, the emotions felt, and the thoughts evoked to accomplish the activity all provide insight into the therapist's role in treatment as a change agent while revealing the potential for the client's own problem-solving abilities.

As stated by Betty Risteen Hasselkus in *The Meaning of Everyday Occupation*, "In occupational therapy, we as therapists have unending opportunities for creative moments in our work. Every client whom we see is unique; every treatment plan we develop and carry out is unique; every time we engage in clinical reasoning, we are using our creative energies to make sense out of the many elements of each new clinical situation" (Hasselkus, 2011, p. 173). Through completing each chapter in succession, the student has the potential to recognize and experience that flow firsthand. This is an important aspect of developing therapeutic use of self and therapeutic use of activity in treating clients. The text provides a variety of ways for eliciting a creative response in the student for envisioning treatment intervention and promoting the client's adaptive response. When occupation is seen as active engagement (what people do), students recognize the uniqueness of how each person's body, mind, and emotions work in concert when performing activities within any occupation. Planning treatment is a creative synthesis of activity analysis with the client's occupational performance skills and patterns, specific personal factors, and the context/environment in which performance takes place (American Occupational Therapy Association, 2008).

Within each chapter, students have opportunities to articulate a rationale, design strategies for accomplishing tasks, and modify theoretical ideas to meet specific criteria. Students also learn to contribute interprofessionally as members of a health care team while working with their peers. By searching for alternative ways to complete assignments, students become aware of the difference between their own learning and working styles through adjusting to those with different ones. This mimics what occurs in practice in identifying the context and environment in which occupation occurs and then discovering what approach will best engage each client in his or her own therapy. Intervention in this creative manner enlists clients as active agents in their own healing. Whether a student, therapist, or client, creativity plays a part in what drives every person's behavior repertoire. Creativity is a resource residing within every person to be called upon to find a different way, see another avenue, or explore a new alternative.

Occupational therapy practitioners plan therapeutic intervention to be a creative engagement in occupation. To help students build these professional skills is the purpose of this text.

References

American Occupational Therapy Association. (2008). Occupational therapy practice framework: Domain & process (2nd ed.). *American Journal of Occupational Therapy, 62*(6), 625-683.

Hasselkus, B. R. (2011). *The meaning of everyday occupation* (2nd ed.). Thorofare, NJ: SLACK Incorporated.

Lamport, N. K., Coffey, M. S., & Hersch, G. I. (1996). *Activity analysis and application: Building blocks of treatment.* Thorofare, NJ: SLACK Incorporated.

Benefits of Creativity:
Building Professional Skills

Defining/identifying creativity

Recognizing/acknowledging use of creativity in OT

Describing the cognitive process of creativity

Understanding the neuroscience and structures of creativity

Incorporating creativity into professional skills

Applying creativity in client intervention

Applying research in creativity

1

Perceptions of Creativity

Nancy K. Lamport, MS, OTR

OBJECTIVES

1. Recognize that the ability to be creative is present throughout one's life.
2. Understand some common definitions of creativity.
3. Identify creative potential as an aspect of thinking and problem solving.

UNIT 1: CREATIVITY

Creativity is a nebulous entity. What is it? Where does it come from? Who has it? Who does not? Are we born with it? Can it be developed? Can it be discouraged? Or, worse yet, can it be erased? Does it require a certain kind of intelligence? What is the difference between creativity and ingenuity? How would the topic of creativity relate to becoming an occupational therapy practitioner?

In this chapter, some current ways of defining creativity are provided, and the latent creativity present at birth and fostered throughout human development is explored. How this creative capacity enters our social, interactive, and problem-solving skill set is recognized as a disappearing trait that can reappear as needed.

When random people on the street are questioned about their creative abilities, some might say "I don't have any creativity; I can't draw a straight line with a ruler." Creativity in arts and crafts, theater performances, dance recitals, and music concerts is easy to see. The facility of words by writers, playwrights, and poets is also readily apparent. Many professionals depend on their creativity to extend productivity in their chosen work. Some of them have undergone specific education to enhance their potential and capability to solve problems creatively. Others appear to have a talent for instinctively expressing creativity in their approach to everyday life. Do people learn creativity through their education, or do they express and exhibit a natural creativity that comes from within them?

There will always be people who depend on their creativity to live as painters, artists, authors, musicians, architects, educators, engineers, explorers, landscape designers, city planners, and inventors. They see the big picture and/or small details and have an accompanying ability to manipulate materials, spaces, and rules through their endeavors that can build communities, promote culture, develop medical procedures, pursue research, and provide an understanding of world responsibilities. Do all persons have creative capacity within them that can be tapped as well?

Coffey MS, Lamport NK, Hersch GI.
Creative Engagement in Occupation: Building Professional Skills (pp 1-7).
© 2015 SLACK Incorporated.

One of the barriers in identifying personal creativity is discounting the everyday creativity within our daily lives. A young child inventing a new game using stuffed toys, a sheet, and a card table opens up an imaginary animal hospital. A mother turns leftover items in the refrigerator into an original food combination that makes an appealing meal. These are examples of creativity that one can see in everyday life. Many people have a need to express their creativity by repeating daily tasks in new or novel ways, such as driving home using a different route than taken to get to work or displaying family pictures on a mantel with their favorite objects and mementos. They may lose interest in the drive or the room if they cannot vary the conditions under which they experience them. Is this creativity or just a burst of initiative that mimics true creativity?

Unit 2: Identification of the Impact of Creativity Over Time

The origin and development of creativity are difficult to pinpoint. If one has had the privilege of observing young children from birth through their preschool years, it may be easy to observe when creativity appears. In this period of early childhood, there are innumerable experiences that stimulate the senses, encourage physical and mental growth, and provide experimental and practice arenas for a child to fit into the fabric of family and social interaction. The battle cry is, "What is it? What can I do with it? Will it break? Where can I put it? Will a blue one do the same thing as a red one? Why are there square ones and round ones? Will it hurt? How high can I climb? What do you mean by 'share'?"

Most children run; they do not walk. They are so eager to get from one activity to the next that walking takes too long. They squirm and shout, jump and tumble in their efforts to try out as much of their world as they can between dawn and sunset, and sometimes long after that. Even at this early age, it is possible to identify a sense of joy in their creative, unstructured play. Their inner spark of inquisitiveness gives them the confidence they need to explore, even at their own peril. Parents must teach safety first because their children's insight and inhibition are poorly developed at this stage.

Then, the school bell rings and the school doors close, followed by at least 12 and maybe more years of prescriptive learning, obeying the rules, lining up, coloring within the lines, seeking praise for the right answers, and encountering shame for too many of the wrong ones.

Exercise in the gym, peer pressure, homework, sports, scouts, and quick dinners before practice interfere with previously spontaneous endeavors. Independent thinking, initiative, and discovery may suffer and disappear as time constraints and energy are diverted into other channels. So may long walks with family, the discovery of a seashell's song when placed to an ear, reading books with a friend under a tree, or pondering where a flock of geese flying overhead may be going. Creativity may take a back seat to expected solutions to assignments, as aptitudes are measured by standardized tests with only one answer to each question.

After high school, more prescriptive schooling may come with college, trade school, apprenticeships, or military service. Young adults begin careers, fall in love, and start a family. They may finance a car, a house, or braces for young teeth while balancing credit card debt and juggling work, home, school, church, and social schedules; not much time for unbridled creativity here. Or is there? All these events require planning, organization, and time management for life tasks they have never experienced. The new roles assumed as spouse, parent, or worker and the responsibilities accrued during young adulthood are preparation for experiences in middle adulthood. In these middle years, a change of job or career ambition or adult children returning home to attend to the needs of parents who encounter disabling health issues can arise. Are making adjustments, coping, and taking one day at a time doing what is necessary? Or, is this where creativity once again plays an active role and takes center stage?

Then comes a third period of the human experience: retirement. In the United States, retirement is viewed as a stage of life that one has earned or deserves regardless of whether the means to achieve it is possible. Up until that time, most people are identified to themselves and to others by what they do in their personal realms of employment, family, friends, and community. When the massive door that led to daily work obligations closes and the flimsy door that leads to retirement opens, is there a broad, seemingly endless, and unmarked open path on the other side? What will the pass through this unchartered territory mean to the adult who crosses the threshold? What will it mean to the significant others involved? How will the person's role as a retiree be defined, and what meaningful activities will there be?

For some, this door opens slowly, sometimes more than once, and provides time to develop a new identity and purpose. For others, the door may be opened by the strong wind of circumstance, leaving little time to think about what might be ahead. In either case, creative planning can be the means to a successful retirement regardless of circumstances. Both mental health and optimum function are dependent on operative answers to issues regarding available resources, current family and financial responsibilities, health costs, and living conditions. Will this path of opportunities be nourished by the person's innate creativity, or will it be one of unknowns, indecision, lack of initiative, and discouragement? All facets of society in general, and the practice of occupational therapy in particular, provide the opportunity to consider answers in these areas with the rapidly expanding mature population. To foster and achieve productive aging requires creative problem solving for a population that is increasing with each generation.

Downsizing, reprioritizing needs, locating new resources, and desiring to undertake different activities can shift values and change decisions about pursuing some life tasks.

Once again, the wheels of exploration need to be put into motion. Creative contemplation of each individual's goals for retirement must be defined. Is this the time for entertaining daydreams about accomplishments one has longed to attain and seeking the opportunities to achieve them? Daily activities need to be identified, priorities set, and chosen tasks completed so that at the end of the day, one may look back at positive accomplishments (e.g., "I made something for the bake sale at church. I learned a new way to compile recipes on the computer. I helped someone connect with my financial planner at a seminar. I played a good game of tennis at the gym. I ate lunch and had a good talk with a friend. I jotted down important memories and wrote a poem about them. I volunteered in a community project for the food pantry. I helped a neighbor child fly his kite. I worked on my plans to go to Spain.") These examples illustrate how the individual purposefully chooses to create meaningful activities outside his or her previous roles and routines.

Unit 3: Creativity Defined

Definitions of creativity are many and diverse, depending on the terms of the discipline that is defining it. Anthony Brandt (2011), Artistic Director of a contemporary music ensemble and Associate Professor at Rice University's Shepherd School of Music, sees creativity as an underlying mechanism in our mental lives. He asserts that our brains operate using two types of behavior—automated and mediated—both of which are needed for human development. The automated behavior denotes reliability and mediation, requiring rote memorization, repetitive practice, and responses to questions that have one answer. No exploration is attempted, and only the right answers are to be found and given. Mediated behavior, however, requires flexibility and the ability to keep an open mind. This behavior is characterized

by a synthesis with subjective reasoning and arriving at questions for which there is no single correct response. Instead, a new answer to meet the moment is the goal. The role of the arts is important in encouraging and developing this type of thinking.

Brandt (2011) refers to a unified model of creativity proposed by cognitive scientists Mark Turner and Gilles Fauconnier, which states that creativity involves an alteration of some kind. Brandt proposes three types of alteration: bending, breaking, and blending. In his theory, *bending* involves transforming the original idea. *Breaking* occurs when the original idea is altered beyond recognition. *Blending* occurs when these two sources are merged. As an example, in music, bending is a variation on a theme, breaking is fragmenting or contrasting the theme, and blending becomes a counterpoint. He recognizes that the human brain is constantly choosing to automate or mediate and is unique in the animal world. Without constant use of both facets, brain function is diminished. From Brandt's perspective, the inclusion of the arts throughout the educational process is necessary for all human beings to ensure competence in both types of behavior.

The role of creativity has been used to explain how *Homo sapiens* gained the edge to survive when other species died out as a result, in part, of the lack of this phenomenon. Current concepts suggest that creativity is the prerogative of people with artistic abilities who are talented in art, music, writing, or theater.

However, consider those who enjoy developing new ideas in their area of personal interest or in a social program in their community. Cohen (2000), in his book *The Creative Age*, views creativity as a process and an inner resource within every human being. As Founder and Director of the Washington, D.C., Center on Aging, he sees this process as an important aspect of being engaged throughout our lives, helping to develop our potential and envision challenges as opportunities. Other aspects that enhance this quality may be the context and environment in which we live or the influence of our individual personalities, such as an active imagination or persistence in the midst of obstacles. Our creativity may surface, then submerge and reappear at a later time, and we each have it available to be called upon when needed (p. 19).

Cohen (2000, p. 169) makes reference to psychologist Howard Gardner who clarifies these phases with a simple but encompassing definition in which he divides creativity into two categories: creativity with a "big C" and creativity with a "little c."

Creativity with a "big C" applies to the extraordinary accomplishments of unusual or gifted people. These forms of creativity not only change entire fields of thought but also influence other fields and, in some ways, world history. Creativity with a "little c" is grounded in various and sundry realities of life. Every person has certain areas in which he or she has special abilities.

In a later book entitled *The Mature Mind*, Cohen (2005) describes four life phases in psychological development during the second half of life. He begins with a midlife evaluation of where one has been, who one is now, and where one is going that takes place within the 40- to 65-year age group. The liberation phase overlaps midlife and spans years 60 to 70, when individuals seek freedom from earlier limitations and inhibitions while their brain is undergoing physiological changes and sprouting new connections. The result is a more balanced use of both hemispheres as one ponders, "if not now, when?" In the late 60s to 80s, a desire to give back to family, friends, and society is coupled with a continuing desire to go on, despite adversity or loss. Apparently, people remain vital with new manifestations of creativity and social engagement up to the end of life. In fact, they may become more powerfully motivated and energized with new direction or purpose (Cohen, 2005, pp. 52-53). Cohen calls the fuel of impelling force of inner drives, urges, and desires that wax and wane throughout our life "[t]he inner push" (p. 32).

Therese Schmid is an Australian occupational therapist who developed the following definition from her research on health through creativity:

> Creativity is the innate capacity to think and act in original ways, to be inventive, to be imaginative and to find new and original solutions to needs, problems, and forms of expression. It can be used in all activities. Its processes and outcomes are meaningful to its user and generate positive feelings. (Schmid, 2005, p. 6)

Schmid views creativity as an intrinsic part of the philosophy of occupational therapy, and she is not alone. Pierce (2003), in her book entitled *Occupation by Design: Building Therapeutic Power*, emphasizes the importance of and demand for the creative skills of occupational therapy practitioners in every area of practice as a daily occurrence (p. 264). She envisions treatment in which each therapist creates an individual "balance of occupations by blending the characteristics of productivity, pleasure, and restoration" (p. 33). Tessa Perrin (2001), an occupational therapist in Essex, Great Britain, sees the "creativity of [the] therapeutic relationship" as central to health and well-being and the successful outcome dependent upon the "liberating aspect of creativity" within it (p. 131). In this respect, the ability to be creative in working with clients can be one of the reasons occupational therapy initially attracts students to enter the profession (Hasselkus, 2011, p. 174).

UNIT 4: RELATED RESEARCH

A Snapshot

Cohen's four phases of psychological development (2005, pp. 52-54) appear to be closely matched by the women in a middle-class neighborhood support group to which this author (Lamport) belonged. Lamport used an informal questionnaire to explore how their lives had changed in the past 10 years, including their sense of identity and the influence of creative thinking on their outlook. She directed the discussion during one of the early sessions of this ongoing support group as a way for group members to become acquainted with each other. All of the participants were more than 50 years of age, several were retired, and their health was rated as good overall, without reference to existing medical conditions.

A definition of creativity from Wikipedia was used and a distinction made between innovation (the process of generating and applying creative ideas) and creativity to open the discussion.

The questions she asked were as follows:

1. As you have gotten older, what are you doing now that you did not do 10 years ago?

2. Is the ability to be creative important to you?

3. Is time a factor in your interest in being creative?

4. Do you see yourself in the process of adopting a new identity?

5. Do you notice that creative thinking influences this new outlook?

Being known by what we do was the perception of one's identity before retirement took place, and some of the women were content with who they were. Some had experienced notable life changes in the past 10 years, such as the loss of a spouse, a new marriage, an increase in family size due to marriage, and the addition of grandchildren. The ability to be creative in both public and personal endeavors was expressed as important to each person. The retired women especially valued the time that was now theirs to volunteer, read, sew, quilt, or garden. Having time to explore a new hobby, craft, or art activity was a joy. Adequate time to develop organization within their lives helped provide peace of mind, especially in family matters in which grandmotherly duties constantly called for their attention. In the public sector, several women were leaders in an organization focusing on procuring and dispensing clothing and school supplies for children. One woman was the president of a group that recruited neighbors to participate as volunteers. Several women had leadership roles in church activities, book clubs, and neighborhood events, such as the yearly picnic and the sponsoring of art classes. All of them were involved with some type of philanthropy with their families or in public organizations.

An interesting sidelight was that none of the women thought of themselves as particularly creative, despite the obvious evolution of their lives in terms or roles, routines, and renewal over the past decade. The consensus was that what they did and how they went about living their lives were just expressions of the "way we were." Creativity was a problem-solving mechanism for them, as it is for many people, but was not thought of as a separate entity enlisted for making these quite visible life transitions. Several women said that they were "not creative."

UNIT 5: ACKNOWLEDGING AND ACCESSING YOUR OWN CREATIVITY

To recognize that creativity is an inherent and useful part of their lives, people must recognize its impact and the possibilities within themselves. In recent years, employees have been looking for workers who can generate new ideas and processes that expand their efforts beyond their job description. In other words, creative people who can use the combination of intellect and training with their particular skills to further outcomes in the workplace are sought and hired.

Consider the electronic explosion in diverse areas that has occurred during the past 10 years. The Apple iPad is certainly the conscious use and application of creativity, but so is the use of the iPad as a therapeutic tool in occupational therapy. To enlist the iPad as a viable way to improve motor skills, engage sensory and visual perception, or enhance communication and social participation to meet identified goals is being creative. The invention of the iPad is one example of the "big C" concept. The ability to configure the iPad in evidence-based practice or to increase work productivity, network professionally, or educate through creative use of this product in coursework is an example of the "little c" concept. The iPad itself is being used as "ground" for fostering new skills and to generate purposeful activity.

To further explore your own creativity, Worksheets 1-1 and 1-2 are included to prompt further reflection on your life at this point in time. Use them as jumping-off points to stimulate your interest in discovering when and how you engage creatively.

CONCLUSION

Ideas and definitions about creativity have been introduced in this chapter as a starting point for understanding the role of creativity in occupational therapy. An innate ability to be creative is present in every individual, whether student, client, or practitioner. Identifying the creative aspects inherent in living from day to day is important in recognizing how a person performs in meaningful areas of occupation. The important roles to fill, the past experiences that influence present capabilities, and the possible avenues for future achievement are all aspects of treatment intervention. Creativity is a component of this process with an unknown potential to change the outcomes.

QUESTIONS

1. How has this chapter changed your understanding of creativity?

2. Can you distinguish between creativity and ingenuity?

3. What levels and/or types of creativity do you identify in yourself? In other people you know?

4. In defining creativity, how important is a new outcome? Why or why not?

5. Are the types of creativity we exhibit different depending on our age? Why or why not?

REFERENCES

Brandt, A. (2011, September 7). For sake of society, young minds need art. *Houston Chronicle.* Retrieved from http://www.chron.com/opinion/outlook/article/For-sake-of-society-young-minds-need-art-2159859.php.

Cohen, G. D. (2000). *The creative age.* New York, NY: Harper-Collins.

Cohen, G. D. (2005). *The mature mind.* New York, NY: Basic Books.

Hasselkus, B. (2011). *The meaning of everyday occupation.* Thorofare, NJ: SLACK Incorporated.

Perrin, T. (2001). Don't despise the fluffy bunny: A reflection from practice. *British Journal of Occupational Therapy, 64*(3), 132.

Pierce, D. (2003). *Occupation by design: Building therapeutic power.* Philadelphia, PA: F. A. Davis.

Schmid, T. (Ed.). (2005). *Promoting health through creativity.* Philadelphia, PA: Whurr Publishing.

Worksheet 1-1

Creative Outlets in My Life

Check all of the following activities you are currently performing:

_____ I like to doodle, draw, or color pictures.

_____ I make items for myself or other people as gifts.

_____ I take different routes to travel to my destination (by foot, bicycle, car, train, boat, plane).

_____ I enjoy looking at picture books or taking pictures (camera, phone, iPad).

_____ I send e-cards or handwritten notes with personal messages to friends/family.

_____ I hang pictures on my wall or bulletin board of _____ people _____ places _____ events important to me.

_____ I own something that I love to look at but has no real use or value to others.

_____ I explore places to see what's new, such as a zoo, shopping mall, library, restaurant, museum, specialty store, or art gallery.

_____ I collect one-of-a-kind items or have a collection I consider important to me personally.

_____ I own things from family members who have died that I consider worthy of being saved.

_____ I watch for new events to attend, such as festivals, fairs, or exhibits.

_____ I go to places where artists sell their creative work or vendors have unique items for sale.

_____ I enter my own creative work in the county fair, contests, or other competitions.

_____ I display my own/family member's creative work in a place where I can view it frequently.

_____ I notice the way buildings, such as houses, stores, and offices, differ from each other.

_____ I attend a church, temple, mosque, or house of faith to contemplate, worship, or participate in activities.

_____ I stop to read the inscriptions on monuments, gravesites, or sculptures.

_____ I scrapbook, make photo albums, jot down family stories, or do genealogy work.

_____ I take walks, visit parks, hike, backpack, camp, or travel to locations to see their natural beauty.

List a minimum of 3 items for each of the following:

I want to continue doing:	I would like to try doing:	I also do the following:
1.	1.	1.
2.	2.	2.
3.	3.	3.

Worksheet 1-2

Creativity Questionnaire

Make note of the first thoughts and feelings that come to mind when you read the statements below. Be prepared to share these with other students in a small group discussion.

1. Creativity is often defined as the process of generating new ideas or associations of existing ideas or concepts. It also may be defined as the act of taking something and making it into something else.

    a. Is the ability to be creative important to you? Why or why not?

    b. Is time a factor in your interest in being creative? Why or why not?

    c. Do circumstances and/or other people define whether you view what you are doing as creative?

    d. How do these factors affect your own perception of being creative?

2. Who we are is often defined by what we do or what others view us doing. These activities can cast us in roles we choose or that others choose for us. Based on what you do as a student, your identity as a student may be viewed as a priority for you. To others, you may be seen primarily as a friend, sibling, spouse, neighbor, employee, or stranger.

    a. What are you doing now that you did not do 5 years ago?

    b. What new identity do you see yourself in the process of adopting?

    c. How does creative thinking influence your ability to change into this new identity?

    d. How will this identity differ from the identity you hold currently?

Benefits of Creativity: Building Professional Skills

Defining/identifying creativity

Recognizing/acknowledging use of creativity in OT

Describing the cognitive process of creativity

Understanding the neuroscience and structures of creativity

Incorporating creativity into professional skills

Applying creativity in client intervention

Applying research in creativity

2

Expressions of Creativity in Occupational Therapy

Margaret S. Coffey, MA, COTA, ROH

In every person's life, where and how one "grew up" influences what and why choices are made to explore different activities. One's culture and environment affect the patterns of behavior, the routines and habits, even the roles taken to perform everyday occupations. People-watching the particular ways others engage in their chosen occupations reveals different points of view and an appreciation for the diversity possible. Observing people can also uncover the creative ways they learn, problem solve, review, resolve, and grow through their experiences.

Events such as making dinner, shopping at the mall, text messaging, or attending a Friday night get-together can be a fascinating enterprise as one begins to "think like an occupational therapist." When the steps taken to complete these everyday tasks are uncovered and made known, the simplest of activities seems filled with purpose. The scope of *how* occupational therapy can benefit an individual unable to perform a meaningful activity is expanded.

Exploring a client's personal history is part of the evaluation process conducted by an occupational therapy practitioner. As a student, integrating the knowledge-base of occupational therapy into one's own history is an important resource for working with clients. As the student develops professional skills, clinical reasoning expands and improves for devising treatment that specifically engages each client in occupational therapy. As a new therapist, the student will partner with the client

to improve, restore, or compensate for the loss or decline of specific skills. Thinking on the part of the practitioner becomes more fluid while being sharpened and polished to meet clients' needs within their context and environment. Providing opportunities for people to discover their own creativity in the therapy process is especially beneficial. The phrase "it depends…" can be a challenge and password to explore the options possible to find answers in difficult scenarios with unknown solutions.

In this chapter, creativity will be examined from three different perspectives: highlighting how occupational therapy practitioners used one activity in creative ways to engage their clients; understanding how the diversity of contexts and environments affect each person; and exploring creative potential while identifying one's own context and environment.

OBJECTIVES

1. Recognize the creative use of one therapeutic activity commonly used in occupational therapy throughout its history.

2. Understand how context and environment affect clients receiving occupational therapy.

3. Engage in creative experiences while defining one's own context and environment.

Coffey MS, Lamport NK, Hersch GI.
Creative Engagement in Occupation: Building Professional Skills (pp 9-38).
© 2015 SLACK Incorporated.

UNIT 1: ONE ASPECT OF CREATIVITY IN THE HISTORY OF OCCUPATIONAL THERAPY

Occupational therapy became a viable profession during the early 20th century in the midst of significant world events. A brief look at some of these happenings helps provide a context for the appearance of one activity commonly used in occupational therapy treatment.

In 1918, thousands of American soldiers who had been fighting abroad on World War I (WWI) battle-fronts were returning home. At the same time, millions of immigrants continued to flood into the country looking for work, increasing the proportion of different ethnic populations and the size of cities. Economic shifts in the labor force and poor working conditions led to large-scale strikes (Zinn, 2003). Mechanized production techniques had already significantly changed how the individual worker was engaged in occupation (Pierce, 2003). Many of those skilled in crafting items one at a time were now employed in huge industries where the individual was anonymous.

A shift in attitude of the American people began to emerge. Disillusionment, death, and disease meant adapting to a new environment and compensating for the deficits in order to survive. Personal values and meaningful occupation were being reconfigured and redefined for families, a process spanning several generations. The philosophy, art, and political reform occurring during this time accompanied by the rising growth in urban populations and sociological changes reflected this shift (Walford, 2002). Against this backdrop and within this setting, occupational therapy in America developed into a profession.

Disabled servicemen were being brought into hospitals and asylums for convalescence with psychological damage as well as physical trauma (Quiroga, 1995). During the war, the United States recruited and trained reconstruction aides for serving the returning soldiers needing psychiatric and physical rehabilitation. The official description of this work by the Surgeon General's Office was for a "purely medical function for the therapeutic benefit of activity to be prescribed in the early stages of convalescence" in an effort "to occupy [and] prevent hospitalization; to prepare the mind for subsequent occupational [vocational] treatment…and the work to be simple, quickly done, and have commercial value" (Crane, n.d., p. 58).

One of the first skills taught to recruits in the Class B category of aides was the craft of hand weaving. To qualify for these positions, they took a preliminary curriculum that included training in "weaving—in hand and bead looms, simple rug and mat making" (Crane, n.d., p. 59). As a craft, weaving offered the client both a creative dimension and concrete evidence of the ability to affect one's immediate environment. Once learned, the aide could incorporate weaving into treatment even when the patient had no experience in arts and crafts. Weaving activities employed the use of the major performance skills and could provide an expressive outlet for communicating with others (Breines, 1995, p. 55). Over time, weaving activities also proved to provide benefits to a wide range of people in terms of gender, age, ethnicity, and culture. Therapeutic goals could be set individually and suited for a multitude of common diagnoses.

These activities could also be tailored to address the patient's change in status and provide the "just right challenge" through grading. Variables included the amount of energy used, duration and timing of individual steps, number of repetitions of specific movements, and amount of strength required to perform them. The type of equipment used could be sized, such as the portability of stick-weaving or a hand-held frame, to work on a table surface in the recreation area or floor loom in the clinic. Positioning of the equipment in a horizontal or vertical orientation, bedside, or wheelchair height was also possible.

The specific weaving technique offered opportunities for fine and gross motor skills such as precise manipulation while weaving with cards or larger movements using shuttles to hold yarn while weaving on a tapestry loom. The scope of the project undertaken could be limited in the time it took to complete and the size of the product (e.g., small and quick in making a potholder on a square metal frame or large and lengthy as weaving yardage to be made into a garment).

Weaving activities also engaged the client in creative ways. Art techniques and design principles were incorporated through color choice and yarn selection to produce the texture and pattern of the cloth. The technique and objects used in the process could be matched to the cognitive ability and emotional regulation skills of the individual. Weaving as therapy could result in decorative or utilitarian products and held the potential for reflecting the patient's choices through every step of the process.

Mary Meigs Atwater, a volunteer trained as a reconstruction aide near the end of WWI, used weaving activities extensively in treatment, drawing on her own expertise. She saw that the sense of touch was crucial to helping a soldier's return to mental health. "What we think we see or think we hear may be illusion," she stated, " but we never doubt the reality of what we feel with our fingers or hold in our hands" and that it was "chiefly through the hands that the occupational therapist works" (Retter & Patterson, 1992, pp. 148-149). She wrote a correspondence course of instruction "for occupational therapists and students of occupational therapy" including weaving techniques "found useful for ward-work with bed-patients" in her publication of the *Shuttle Craft Guild Bulletin*. In 1943, Atwater, still working in occupational therapy, wrote *Card Weaving in the Practice of Occupational Therapy*, prepared for the use of hospital aides (Tidball, 1952).

During World War II, weaving continued to be an instrumental activity taught and provided in occupational therapy. Wilma West (n.d.) cited its use for orthopedic conditions to increase shoulder flexion, for peripheral nerve injuries to regain strength and movement in hands and fingers, and for upper extremity plastic surgery. Weaving might progress "from gross to fine thread as well as in the motions required by the size of looms and from simple to complex in pattern" and, for the blind, a "Braille type was made by map tacks on a strip of cardboard" (West, n.d., p. 321). Grading the activity or adapting the equipment was common to address the needs of the patient.

When the *Standards for Courses of Training in Occupational Therapy* were drawn up in 1923, the number of hours in textiles was 210 and included weaving with occupational therapy analysis and adaptation (Quiroga, 1995). They focused on the meaning a task held for the individual to be as important to the client as the overall outcome. The underlying assumption of treatment was for the therapist to establish meaningful relationships to motivate positive responses in therapy and is still held today.

By the time both World Wars were over, weaving was accepted as an essential component of occupational therapy education. Mary Black, an OTR who directed weaving instructors in occupational therapy, published *New Key to Weaving* in 1945. When the second edition of her text appeared in 1958, she wrote about using weaving as treatment in the psychiatric hospital. By grading the process, those experiencing poor concentration could be engaged, an awareness of their surroundings awakened, destructive energy redirected, and overactive patients quieted (Black, 1958).

In the professional literature from 1947 to 1965, the ingenuity of therapists using weaving in treatment is clearly documented. It is found in 23 articles appearing in the *American Journal of Occupational Therapy*, ten of them published from 1954 to 1964. Twenty-two of the articles dealt with modification of existing, commercially available equipment and detail the creative approach therapists took to meet their patients' needs through weaving as purposeful activity. Sixteen were listed under the subject heading "Equipment, Therapeutic: Crafts and Work Activities" in *The Twenty-Five Year Cumulative Index of the American Journal of Occupational Therapy*, edited by Cordelia Myers (1973).

The focus of each article was the adaptation of a loom used in treatment warranted by individual patient needs. Changes made to equipment were described, many illustrated with drawings or photographs. Construction notes and operation instructions were often given. The weaving techniques and treatment goals were stated, primarily to improve physical function through offering graded resistance or assistance to the patient. Diagnostic categories included spinal cord injuries, hemiplegia, brachial plexus paralysis, cerebral palsy, poliomyelitis and ischemic myositis, weak ankle dorsiflexors, and amputations. Postoperative cases such as muscle transplants, neuromuscular and metabolic disorders resulting in functional loss of joint motion, arthritis, and hand injuries are also documented. Patients confined to bed in prone or supine positions and those who were ambulatory were mentioned. Original ideas were shared for changing the equipment or tools to provide resistance, isolate movements and muscle function, or permit one-handed instead of two-handed use. The articles also state that weaving was used in treating primary or secondary psychiatric conditions such as depression. Its use in vocational and physical rehabilitation, long-term care facilities, sheltered workshops, psychiatric hospitals, and outpatient clinics is given as well.

In the classroom and the clinic, weaving as a therapeutic activity was further supplemented by the manufacture of a "Rehabilitation Loom" by Bailey Manufacturing Company. Designed for use in occupational therapy curriculums and hospital departments, this floor loom featured a beater bar weight to add resistance and an optional set-up from horizontal to vertical placement of the treadles. An instruction pamphlet included a section specifically addressing the resistive uses of the loom as a "treatment tested" piece of equipment (Bailey Manufacturing, n.d.). In 1971, the Department of the Army was conducting a course entitled *Craft Techniques in Occupational Therapy* with detailed instruction and drawings for learning weaving techniques to be used in treatment.

Twenty years later, the decline of weaving activities in occupational therapy is evident as newer techniques and treatment practices gained precedence. Drake gives a rationale and history of this change when describing the therapeutic use of crafts and the few weaving activities still being used (Drake, 1999, pp. 5, 129-130). Breines indirectly suggests this when she encourages students to learn unfamiliar crafts "used as clinical tools since the profession of occupational therapy was established"

(Breines, 1995, p. 55). Though weaving activities were used throughout the history of occupational therapy, today's treatment context and environment has made them insignificant. Retired occupational therapy practitioners who learned to weave in their professional training often continue this as a hobby for its therapeutic as well as productive benefits. Atwater continued her dedication to weaving and occupational therapy until the day of her death in 1956. Her daughter says at that time she was "working with a neighbor boy who had a damaged hand, using card-weaving, knotting, inkle-loom weaving and braiding to encourage him to regain the use of his hand—and she was succeeding well" (Retter & Patterson, 1992, p. 201).

Within the appropriate context and environment, the talent and resourcefulness of therapists used weaving activities to engage the client in meaningful occupation. Occupational therapy is richer for this heritage. Recreating a time line of the use of weaving in occupational therapy was one way to uncover its potential and success as an activity in treatment. Assignment 2-1 is designed for you to discover your own context and environment through creation of a personal timeline. Perhaps you will see a thread woven into your history with the possibility of helping you as a future therapist.

Assignment 2-1

This assignment is designed for you to discover your personal history through creation of a timeline. In addition to exploring your past, the information shared will be used in a later assignment in this chapter. See Worksheet 2-1 for the complete instructions.

Unit 2: Environment and Context as Keys to Occupational Performance

Imagine what changes will occur for someone as a newly credentialed occupational therapy practitioner starting that first job. From the moment this person gets up in the morning until he or she dives under the covers that night, daily activities may be arranged quite differently from those experienced the previous day. Consider that all of one's performance patterns may undergo change: the *routine* of a quick bite before class in lieu of skipping breakfast altogether to be on time to work; the *habit* of stopping at a drive-through for a pick-me-up beverage on the way to school replaced with

carrying a filled thermos to work; the *pattern of behavior* used in deciding where to take a break between classes compared with visiting the break room between clients; the *role* taken by clocking the number of hours in an online classroom contrasted with the number of therapy sessions provided in the clinic; and the bedtime hour to study for a test replaced with preparing for tomorrow's expected caseload.

The context in which this imaginary person participates in occupation is as important as the environment. The terms *context* and *environment* are used here as defined in the *Third Edition* of *Occupational Therapy Practice Framework: Domain and Process* (OTPF) (American Occupational Therapy Association [AOTA], 2014, p. 542). *Context* relates to the components influencing a person's success in everyday occupational performance, including such reference points as the cultural, personal, physical, social, temporal, and virtual aspects of behavior. *Environment* describes the setting in which the person lives and moves on a daily basis, including the physical and social influences affecting this behavior.

Assignment 2-2

Using your imagination, take one of the roles and activities in the scenario comparing the student with a newbie practitioner and write how you would perform this activity in 10 steps or less.

1. Compare notes with a peer who chose the same task. What differs between you and the other individual's details?

2. In analyzing the performance of this activity, you also need to account for the environment in which it takes place. How does the classroom vs the work setting change the expectation for how the activity is accomplished?

3. Consider the cultural and personal aspects of your own context using the *OTPF* for definitions and discuss them with your peers. In what ways did these aspects influence how you would perform the activity?

Occupational therapy's practice today includes entry into schools, community programs, wellness clinics, hospice care, and outpatient behavioral health settings as well as the traditional setting in hospitals, rehabilitation, and long-term care facilities. There is an emphasis on evidenced-based practice and producing functional outcomes. Purposeful activity and meaningful occupation continue as primary treatment goals with concentration on visible, tangible results for the client.

However, return to health may now be a byproduct of careful discharge planning implemented after leaving treatment. The benefits of receiving occupational therapy often continue for the client long after discharge and not witnessed by the therapist. The creative engagement in occupation taking place in the clinic may become the roadmap for maintaining wellness upon return to home.

Recognition and identification of a person's lifestyle is valuable information to use in designing treatment activities. If all activities used in occupational therapy are to be purposeful, then how the client spends time is a key to understanding what will motivate active participation in treatment. Identifying how time is used by clients provides insight into the context and environment where they engage in their occupations.

ASSIGNMENT 2-3

Complete a time-use instrument called an *Occupational Configuration* on yourself using Worksheet 2-2. As you work on this assignment, make further notes about your context and environment that you began in Assignment 2-1. This time, consider the temporal, virtual, and physical aspects that influence how you spend your time (for definitions and examples, see the *OTPF* [AOTA, 2014, p. 528]).

UNIT 3: OCCUPATIONAL PROFILING TO IDENTIFY CONTEXT AND ENVIRONMENT

From the moment Mary Reilly spoke this phrase in her Eleanor Clarke Slagle lecture, she has directed our profession: "That man, through the use of his hands as they are energized by mind and will, can influence the state of his own health" (Reilly, 1962, p. 2). Then, she further asserted, "The logic of occupational therapy rests upon the principle that man has a need to master his environment, to alter and improve it" (Reilly, 1962, pp. 6-7).

Occupational therapy as a profession has recognized the hidden dimensions of activity that can change the downward spiral of failing health to an upward cycle of expectation, hope, and resolution. Estelle Breines saw shaping one's environment into a safe haven as an evolutionary survival skill of being creative. She asserted that creativity involves risk-taking, yet becomes the avenue for discovering meaningful roles and the purpose in life tasks. "Activity is a tool for healing," she stated and "as

such, it is the process and in the process that healing can take place" (Breines, 1995, p. 42).

The role of an occupational therapy practitioner can be to look at clients and envision their potential within to perform the task under consideration. One of the avenues for eliciting this is suggested by Winifred Dunn. She advocates using a strengths-based approach, "facilitating the discovery, embellishment, exploration, and use of the individuals' strengths and resources," then creating options within the person's environment for opportunities to use them. By doing so, she sees the client's ability to reach goals transformed (Dunn, 2012).

Occupational therapy practitioners gather information about clients in different ways; among them is a chart review, skilled observation, and the use of specific assessment tools. Another key to unlocking a client's potential is to construct an *occupational profile* identifying specific wants and needs. What is possible now for the client? What worked successfully in the past? How does the context and environment support or inhibit the client's ability to participate in the occupation?

The purpose of data gathering for the occupational profile is to answer the questions listed in the "Occupational Profile" section of the *OTPF* (AOTA, 2014, p. 513). These include why the person sought services, what changed in the person's ability to perform important activities, and how performance will improve as a result of receiving them. One method for uncovering this information is to conduct an interview with questions designed to reveal the client's thoughts, feelings, and problem-solving abilities. A directed interview can sometimes show how a client responds to everyday situations in a way that may not be evident in formal assessments or casual conversation. The therapist builds rapport and creates trust through word, tone of voice, and body language, while inviting the client to share more than brief answers to questions.

ASSIGNMENT 2-4

To gain experience in collecting information from a peer, follow the directions given for using Worksheet 2-3 to conduct an interview on a peer who, in turn, will interview you. Complete the demographic information on yourself, then give a copy of your Occupational Configuration (Worksheet 2-2) and the interview form to your interviewer. Take turns asking each other the questions so both interviews are completed at the same time. Your answer to a question may help your peer remember something significant when the same question is posed to him or her. As you complete each step of the interview, pay attention to the physical, cognitive, and social skills your peer uses. Make notes of what you observe regarding appearance, body position and parts in use, verbal and nonverbal expressions, and the tone of voice used. This provides additional information regarding the person's function, view point, and emotional regulation skills.

Understanding the person's context and environment is also needed for providing effective client education. Most people have a preferred learning style when exposed to new information. The ability to retain the information is influenced by the type and amount of content to be learned and where the learning takes place. The therapy environment is a major factor affecting the client's ability to receive and process new information. Sensitivity to a person's physical and mental health plays a part in this as well. The therapist's awareness and identification of the ideal location for best demonstrating his or her skills also help provide effective treatment.

The occupational therapy clinic can be the setting to alleviate pain and promote the client's ability to improve performance or prevent it. In providing hope for clients, "one of our unique capabilities as occupational therapists is the provision of opportunities for meaningful doing that can become transforming experiences, thereby creating a belief in possibilities that were thought lost or were never imagined" (Spencer, Davidson, & White, 1997, p. 197).

Defining in depth the client's context and identifying specific components of the environment can direct treatment outcomes. Use of the client's occupational profile can clarify how evidence-based practice took place by providing a comprehensive understanding of why current performance shows improvement. By analyzing this difference, therapists also uncover the "history and experiences, patterns of daily living, interests, values and needs" of this one person at this point in time (AOTA, 2008, p. 649). Documentation of this difference can justify continued therapy or the need for further adaptations to accommodate the client's needs. In composing an occupational profile, the client's priorities become clear through pulling together in succinct comments the unique aspects of the person's entire lifestyle.

ASSIGNMENT 2-5

Using the Occupational Profile on Worksheet 2-4, condense the information you have collected on yourself while reading this chapter. Refer to the *OTPF* (AOTA, 2014) for the definitions of the terms. Note that not all of the information you have learned about yourself may be relevant. Summarize what is important and unique to you in short phrases in each area.

Instilling hope of success in the client and choosing activities that foster it are the vehicle for reversing the downward spiral to an upward one. A synthesis of one's own creativity and the client's potential creativity must take place within the person's context and environment as the therapy process occurs. This awareness of and appreciation for creativity unfolding within the therapeutic relationship is discussed by Tessa Perin, practicing in a mental health treatment arena in Great Britain. "The client is not the recipient of a ready-made solution, but is an active participant in the formulation of a new one…a creative drive towards a new 'product' must be at the heart of every therapeutic intervention" (Perrin, 2001, p. 132). She experiences this dynamic outcome when her know-it-all role is let go to become a collaborator.

ASSIGNMENT 2-6

Imagine you will be receiving occupational therapy treatment from one of your peers for generalized weakness and temporary loss of use of your dominant upper extremity. Be prepared to discuss your results with a peer using the following questions to help guide your discussion.

1. What areas of occupation will be most affected by your diagnosis? In what specific activities do you think you will need assistance? Can you envision how you might change the way you do the activity to accomplish it independently?

2. What information about yourself would be of most help to your peer regarding your present context and environment? If you see a need to change how you function in either of these, what would it be and how would you change it?

3. Therapy will be scheduled 3 times/week for 3 weeks for your condition. What would be the ideal time for you to receive it based on your Occupational Configuration? How would your daily schedule change if you needed to receive therapy before noon on Monday, Wednesday, and Friday? How would you get to therapy if you are unsafe to drive there independently?

4. What aspects of your own creativity are you aware of in answering these questions? Can you identify creativity on the part of your peer while completing this same process?

In the 2005 Eleanor Clarke Slagle lecture, "Embracing Our Ethos, Reclaiming Our Heart," Suzanne M. Peloquin reviewed our profession's beliefs and values to guide its future direction. She stated the emerging view in this way: "We are pathfinders. We enable occupations that heal. We cocreate daily lives. We reach for hearts as well as hands. We are artists and scientists at once. This is our character; this is our genius; this is our spirit" (Peloquin, 2005, p. 617). This approach counters the idea that occupational therapy's past involvement with arts and crafts such as weaving limits the client's ability to be creative. Adopting a life-long learning *process* to provide effective and innovative therapy treatment includes nurturing one's own creativity to benefit the client in two particular ways: eliciting the creative response in clients to solve their own problems, and validating the client's discovery of their own creativity.

Assignment 2-7

Assignment 2-7 is a creative activity for you to complete using information you have collected on a peer. Follow the instructions for Worksheet 2-5 to construct a collage to symbolically represent this person for presentation in class.

Florence Clark portrayed the creative partnership of client and therapist in her 2010 Inaugural Presidential Address when she stated, "In the stories of our clients' lives, we are co-producers and co-directors with them. We do setting and costume design. As if that's not enough, we become actors, playing a supporting role in our client's quest to have a life worth living" (Clark, 2010, p. 851). The verbs used in *OTPF* intervention approaches suggest that just such a creative component is present in every interaction with clients: create/promote, maintain, establish/restore, and modify/compensate (AOTA, 2014).

Creativity and adaptability can form and drive every individual's behavior repertoire. These capacities reside in each person and contribute to the essence of being unique as a human being. Perrin states, "Creativity is of the essence of life itself, and, if we ignore it, we lose something critical to our understanding of life and growth" (Perrin, 2001, p. 131).

The experience of creatively working with peers in school builds a toolbox of ideas through the trials and errors of problem solving. The practice of creatively engaging clients in occupation builds the professional skills of the therapist. In reflecting on her long practice in occupational therapy, Judy Bowen summarized a guiding principle for new practitioners by saying, "We must challenge (clients) to discover their capacities for the next step. To do this, we must enter their process. We must guide and shape out of an awareness of not only their struggles, but our own" (Bowen, 2006, p. 44). Providing opportunities for creativity and entering into them is one of the unique aspects of occupational therapy as a profession.

Conclusion

In this chapter, several premises are identified in the occupational therapy profession. A client is viewed as a whole person and occupations take place within a context and environment significant to each individual. Occupational therapy practitioners perceive the required skills and activities for performing occupations and can creatively grade or adapt activities to benefit the client in performing these skills. Occupational therapy practitioners use and combine knowledge of the client gained through a variety of techniques to produce a comprehensive picture of the person's occupational nature. This knowledge has the potential to design creative intervention with the client as a participant in the process.

Questions

1. What are the reasons you would use or receive health care today? How does this compare to the time in which our profession was conceived in the early 1900s?

2. In what ways does engaging creatively in "occupation" help people maintain wellness? When you recall being creative in an activity of daily living, what did you do?

3. You have completed several assignments in this chapter involving opportunities to be creative. Which did you enjoy the most and the least? What aspects of your performance support how you answered?

4. How do you define the terms *context* and *environment* in your own words? What impact do your present context and environment have on your ability to succeed as a student?

References

American Occupational Therapy Association. (2008). *Occupational therapy practice framework: Domain and process* (2nd ed.). Bethesda, MD: American Occupational Therapy Association.

American Occupational Therapy Association. (2014). *Occupational therapy practice framework: Domain and process* (3rd ed.). Bethesda, MD: American Occupational Therapy Association.

Bailey Manufacturing. (n.d.). *Instruction manual for #650 treatment tested loom.* Lodi, OH: Author.

Black, M. E. (1958). Weaving as therapy. *Shuttle Craft,* 11-14.

Bowen, J. E. (2006). Reflections from the heart: Questions of meaning. *Occupational Therapy Practice, October 9,* 44.

Breines, E. B. (2004). *Occupational therapy: Activities for practice and teaching.* Philadelphia, PA: Whurr Publishing.

Clark, F. (2010). High-definition occupational therapy: HD OT. *American Journal of Occupational Therapy, 64*(6), 848-854.

Crane, A. G. (n.d.). Medical Department of US Army in the World War, Vol. XIII, Retrieved from http://history.amedd.army.mil/booksdocs/wwi/VolXIII/CH02Pt1rev.htm.

Department of the Army. (1971). Craft techniques in occupational therapy. Washington, D.C.: U. S. Government Printing Office.

Drake, M. (1999). *Crafts in therapy and rehabilitation, 2nd edition.* Thorofare, NJ: SLACK Incorporated.

Dunn, W., Blackwell, A., Cox, J., Patten Koenig, K., Pope, E., Sabata, D., & Foster, L. (2012, April). DDSIS annual program: Harnessing strengths—Your Secret weapon for transforming the effectiveness of your practice. Handout at the AOTA Conference, Indianapolis, IN.

Myers, C. (Ed.). (1973). *The twenty-five year cumulative index of the American Journal of Occupational Therapy.* Rockville, MD: American Occupational Therapy Association.

Peloquin, S. M. (2005). Embracing our ethos, reclaiming our heart. *American Journal of Occupational Therapy, 59*(6), 611-625.

Perrin, T. (2001). Don't despise the fluffy bunny: A reflection from practice. *British Journal of Occupational Therapy, 64*(3), 129-134.

Pierce, D. E. (2003). *Occupation by design: Building therapeutic power.* Philadelphia, PA: F. A. Davis Company.

Quiroga, V. A. M. (1995). *Occupational therapy: The first 30 years: 1900 to 1930.* Bethesda, MD: American Occupational Therapy Association.

Retter, M. J. & Patterson, V. (Ed.). (1992). *Weaving a life: The story of Mary Meigs Atwater.* Loveland, CO: Interweave Press.

Reilly, M. (1962). Occupational therapy can be one of the great ideas of 20th century medicine. *American Journal of Occupational Therapy, 16*(1), 1-9.

Spencer, J., Davidson, H., & White, V. (1997). Helping clients develop hopes for the future. *American Journal of Occupational Therapy, 51*(3), 191-198.

Tidball, H. Mary Meigs Atwater: An appreciation. *Handweaver & Caftsman,* Winter 1952-1953, p. 19.

Walford, E. J. (2002). *Great themes in art.* Upper Saddle River, NJ: Prentice-Hall, Inc.

West, W. L. (n.d.). U. S. Army Medical Department, Office of Medical History. Professional Services of Occupational Therapists, World War II

Zinn, H. (2003). *A people's history of the United States.* New York: HarperCollins Publishers.

Worksheet 2-1

Personal Occupational History Project

Part 1

Perform an occupational self-assessment by documenting your own history through constructing a cultural time-line of your life in three or more segments. For example, record your current age and divide it into thirds. If you are 30 years old, the first third is from birth to age 10, the second third from age 11 to age 20, and the final third from age 21 to 30 (your current age). Choose three to five important life events from each segment of your history to briefly describe or highlight. Refer to the *OTPF* (AOTA, 2008) to determine in what area of occupation each event would be placed. Remember that the definition of *occupation* is not about your job but the everyday activities that you perform in your life. Concentrate on the Areas of Occupation, their definitions, and how your life reflects these areas. The end product should be the beginning of a definition of you as an occupational human being.

Illustrate your timeline two-dimensionally in any way you would like—vertically, horizontally, or free-form—to show a time progression. Create your timeline in a way that is easy to read visually, and use words sparingly to identify the transitions from one timeframe to the next. Choose symbols or "frame" the events that mark a change in your life so that it is clear how you perceive a difference or change of direction in your own history.

Part 2

Develop an occupational plan for one area of your life that is not related to becoming an occupational therapy practitioner. Using your timeline as a reference point, figure out where you are, where you want to go, and how you might get there. For example, you may want to raise a family, build your own home, or compete in professional horseback-riding events. Identify an area in one of the occupations from Part 1, and develop a goal statement related to it. List at least three steps you think you must take to achieve it. Record this information on a separate piece of paper to be used in Part 3.

Part 3

You will present your timeline and occupational plan orally to your peers within 3 to 5 minutes. During your presentation, you are to demonstrate an understanding of the *OTPF* areas of occupation and how your culture has influenced your life thus far.

Student Sample 1. Personal Occupational History Project Cultural Lifeline. (Reprinted with permission of Kembe Frederick.)

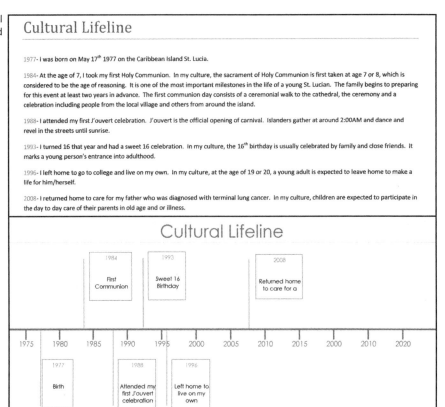

Cultural Lifeline

1977- I was born on May 17th 1977 on the Caribbean Island St. Lucia.

1984- At the age of 7, I took my first Holy Communion. In my culture, the sacrament of Holy Communion is first taken at age 7 or 8, which is considered to be the age of reasoning. It is one of the most important milestones in the life of a young St. Lucian. The family begins to preparing for this event at least two years in advance. The first communion day consists of a ceremonial walk to the cathedral, the ceremony and a celebration including people from the local village and others from around the island.

1988- I attended my first J'ouvert celebration. J'ouvert is the official opening of carnival. Islanders gather at around 2:00AM and dance and revel in the streets until sunrise.

1993- I turned 16 that year and had a sweet 16 celebration. In my culture, the 16th birthday is usually celebrated by family and close friends. It marks a young person's entrance into adulthood.

1996- I left home to go to college and live on my own. In my culture, at the age of 19 or 20, a young adult is expected to leave home to make a life for him/herself.

2008- I returned home to care for my father who was diagnosed with terminal lung cancer. In my culture, children are expected to participate in the day to day care of their parents in old age and or illness.

Student Sample 2. Personal Occupational History Project Cultural Timeline. (Reprinted with permission of Alex Tesmer.)

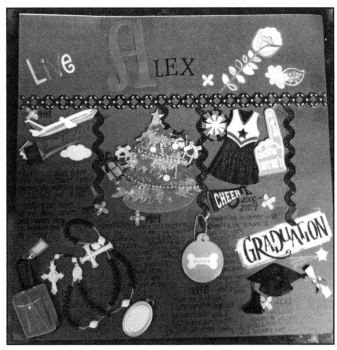

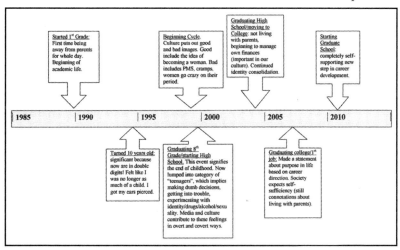

Student Sample 3. Personal Occupational History Project. (Reprinted with permission of Kathryn J. Swope.)

Worksheet 2-2

Occupational Configuration

Name: _____ Interviewed by: _____ Date: _____

List the occupations in which you usually engage during the times specified by referring to what would be an average week's activities. Include subcategories listed in the *OTPF*; also separate study and in-class time, homework, and travel time to/from school.

LATE NIGHT/EARLY MORNING	MONDAY	TUESDAY	WEDNESDAY	THURSDAY	FRIDAY	SATURDAY	SUNDAY
12:00 – 1:00							
1:00 – 2:00							
2:00 – 3:00							
3:00 – 4:00							
4:00 – 5:00							

(continued)

Initials _____

MORNING	MONDAY	TUESDAY	WEDNESDAY	THURSDAY	FRIDAY	SATURDAY	SUNDAY
5:00 – 6:00							
6:00 – 7:00							
7:00 – 8:00							
8:00 – 9:00							
9:00 – 10:00							
10:00 – 11:00							
11:00 – 12:00							

(continued)

Initials _____

AFTERNOON	MONDAY	TUESDAY	WEDNESDAY	THURSDAY	FRIDAY	SATURDAY	SUNDAY
12:00 – 1:00							
1:00 – 2:00							
2:00 – 3:00							
3:00 – 4:00							
4:00 – 5:00							
5:00 – 6:00							

(continued)

Initials _____

EVENING/ NIGHT	MONDAY	TUESDAY	WEDNESDAY	THURSDAY	FRIDAY	SATURDAY	SUNDAY
6:00 – 7:00							
7:00 – 8:00							
8:00 – 9:00							
9:00 – 10:00							
10:00 – 11:00							
11:00 – 12:00							

Worksheet 2-3

Occupational Profile Interview

The intent of this assignment is to gather information about the client and the meaningful roles, performance skills, and areas of occupation that are important to him or her and to establish rapport. The person being interviewed is not required to answer every question and makes the decision about what information he or she wants to share with the interviewer.

Part 1: Demographic Data (circle answers as needed)

Client Name: _____

Birth Date/Age: _____   **Sex:** m   f   **Marital Status:** sin   mar   wid   div   sep

Ethnicity: White   Black   Hispanic   Native American   Asian   Other

Level of Education Completed:

    Elementary school   Junior high school   High school or GED

    Some college   Associate degree   Baccalaureate degree or equivalent

    Master's degree   Doctorate level degree

Residential Situation: _____

_____ **Length of Time in Current Residence:** _____

Others Residing With You: _____

_____

Medical Diagnosis, Condition, or Functional Problem Affecting an Area of Occupation: _____

_____

_____

_____

Medications: _____

Part 2: Questionnaire

1. How would you describe yourself? (What are your strengths and weaknesses? What do you like about yourself? What would you change?) _____

_____

_____

_____

_____

2. What would you say are your current life roles?   student   worker   volunteer   caregiver   home maintainer   friend   family member   religious participant   hobbyist/amateur   organization member   other_____

3. What activities do you *like* to do on a daily basis? Please name them.

_____

_____

_____

_____

_____

4. At what activities do you excel? What physical, mental, or social skills help you?

_____

_____

_____

_____

_____

5. What gives your life meaning or purpose at this point in time?

_____

_____

_____

_____

_____

6. What activities are important to you? What do these activities mean to you? How are they important?

_____

_____

_____

_____

_____

7. Are there any activities you would like to do that, due to major life changes, you cannot?
   If so, what are they? What stops you from participating in these activities? Why would you like to do these activities?

_____

_____

_____

_____

_____

8. What activity would you like to do right now? Why? What meaning does it have for you?

_____

_____

_____

_____

_____

Other Comments or Observations: _____

_____

OT Interviewer: _____   **Date:** _____

Student Sample 4

Sample of Peer Occupational Profile Interview

The intent of this assignment is to gather information about the client and the meaningful roles, performance skills, and areas of occupation that are important to him or her and to establish rapport. The person being interviewed is not required to answer every question and makes the decision about what information he or she wants to share with the interviewer.

Part 1: Demographic Data (circle answers as needed)

Client Name: B.B.

Birth Date/Age: 31   **Sex:** m (f)   **Marital Status:** sin (mar) wid div sep

Ethnicity: White   Black   (Hispanic)   Native American   Asian   Other

Level of Education Completed: *You are currently in school, but what is the highest level of education you have already achieved?*

Elementary school	Junior high school	(High school) or GED
Some college	Associate degree	Baccalaureate degree or equivalent
Master's degree	Doctorate level degree	

Residential Situation: *What kind of living situation do you have?*   Own home   **Length of Time in Current Residence:** *How long have you lived there?*   6 years   **Others Residing With You:**   Children and spouse

What are your major responsibilities while living there?   Household management: laundry, cooking, cleaning, caring for children

Medical Diagnosis, Condition, or Functional Problem Affecting an Area of Occupation: *Do you have any medical conditions or problems that prevent you from performing any activities?*   No, B.B. tries to stay fairly healthy to be able to play and do active things with her kids.

Do you need a prescribed medication to function or address this problem?   Student does not need any medication to function. There are no problems that need to be addressed.

Part 2: Questionnaire

1. *How would you describe yourself? (What are your strengths and weaknesses? What do you like about yourself? What would you change?)*

   Student likes to be organized. She indicates that she has a good memory. However, she is good at forgetting bad things that happen; she referred to events with her former husband. She feels that she truly forgets them unless someone brings them up and triggers her memory. She says she is a good mother and enjoys time with her children.

   B.B. would like to be better organized and manage her time better. She also would like to be more friendly. She says that it seems like people don't like her until they get to know her.

2. *What would you say are your current life roles?*   (student)   worker   (volunteer)   (caregiver)   (home maintainer)   friend   (family member)   (religious participant)   hobbyist/amateur   organization member   other: parent, Sunday school teacher, leader, helper, member in Student Occupational Therapy Association (SOTA) Club, and participant at her church

Which one(s) give you the most satisfaction and why?

Volunteering and teaching at Sunday school give B.B. the most satisfaction because she can see that the kids enjoy it. She also indicates that she gets a lot of satisfaction from spending time with her own kids.

3. *What activities do you like to do on a daily basis (in* addition *to your other responsibilities)? Please name them*

B.B. enjoys running when she has time. She likes walking with her kids to her parents' house, which is in close proximity to her home.

4. *At what activities do you excel?*

Student says, "I am good at cooking." She also indicates that she is good at being a parent. She plays age-appropriate games with each child: hopscotch, jump rope, board games, and Wii.

Student also indicates being good at leading and teaching her Sunday School children. She says that they look forward to the days that it is her turn to teach.

What physical, mental, or social skills help you?

B.B. tries to stay in good physical shape to participate with her kids. She tries to think like her kids to engage well with them. In functioning with her children, she seems to understand "therapeutic use of self." She says she is successful with her Sunday School kids because she is socially "safe" with them. They can trust her, and she makes treats for them. She does not talk about them to other church members in a way that does not respect the privacy of the kids.

5. *Tell me about a situation in which you needed help with something or someone?*

B.B. realized she needed help with her wedding planning, decorating, and food preparation. She indicated that she would have been overwhelmed had it not been for the help of her family members.

How did you get the help you needed?

B.B. asked her mom, sister, and sister-in-law. She knew her sister-in-law was good with decorations and found that she had a lot of good ideas.

6. *What activities are important to you? What do these activities mean to you? How are they important?*

B.B. says that four categories of activities are important to her right now: being there for her kids, cooking and housekeeping, being a Sunday School teacher, and her education. Being active with her kids is important to B.B. She wants to take time for them. This shows them she values them, and it brings her pleasure. Doing well in her schoolwork is also important, and she is trying to learn to be a good time manager to use her days productively.

How do you make time to do these important activities?

B.B. schedules her priorities and trades off time studying with time playing. She indicated that she feels an hour-by-hour manual time planner would help her manage her time better.

7. *Tell me about the goals you have for yourself or your plans for your future?*

B.B.'s main goal at this time is to have a job as a certified occupational therapy assistant. She would also like to be more fit and eat healthier.

Which ones are you currently working on?

She is working on objectives toward becoming certified through the occupational therapy assistant program. She is working on fitness by being active with her kids and maintaining a habit of walking.

Which ones are you not able to work toward right now?

B.B. is not currently prepared to work on eating healthier or changing her food habits.

What needs to happen for you to achieve them?

B.B. suggested that she needs to learn to make a physical time budget and live by it. She stated that she would then schedule time to jog.

8. *What are your favorite activities for relaxation or to have fun?*

   <u>Walk, cook, and play with kids.</u>

   What are you most likely to do whenever you have free time?

   <u>Eat or play Wii with her kids.</u>

Other Comments or Observations: _____

_____

OT Interviewer: <u>L.C.</u>   **Date:** _____

Reprinted with permission of Lauri Chupp.

Worksheet 2-4

Occupational Profile

Student: _____   Date: _____

This profile is designed to gain an overview of one's perspective, occupations, and context/environment, including patterns of daily living, interests, values, and needs. Consult the *OTPF* (AOTA, 2014) for definitions of the terms listed below. You are to summarize significant information for yourself after completing the Occupational Configuration.

OCCUPATIONS	PERSON	CONTEXT/ENVIRONMENT
Areas	*Client Factors*	
Activities of daily living (ADL):	Values:	Cultural:
Instrumental ADL:	Beliefs:	Personal:
Rest and sleep:	Spirituality:	Physical:
Education:	Body functions:	Social:
Work:	Body structures:	Temporal:
Play/leisure:	*Performance Skills* Sensory perceptual skills:	Virtual:
Social participation:	Motor and praxis skills:	*Performance Patterns* Habits:
	Emotional regulation skills:	Routines:
	Cognitive skills:	Roles:
	Communication and social skills:	Rituals:

Student Sample 5

Sample of Peer Occupational Profile

Student Interviewed: <u>B.B.</u>   Interviewer: <u>L.C.</u>

This profile is designed to gain an overview of the client's perspective, occupations, and context/environment, including patterns of daily living, interests, values, and needs. Consult the *OTPF* (AOTA, 2008) for definitions of the terms listed below. You are to summarize significant information your peer has stated and/or you have observed from the interview and the Activity Configuration he or she completed. If there is no specific or relevant information for a category, indicate that you have addressed it in the interview by quoting the response given by the client using quotation marks.

OCCUPATIONS	PERSON	CONTEXT/ENVIRONMENT
Areas	*Client Factors*	
Activities of daily living (ADL): B.B. is independent in all ADL.	Values: B.B. values family and her children. She has religious convictions consistent with her church. She indicates that she understands the importance of setting boundaries with people who relate in unhealthy ways.	Cultural: B.B. has a Hispanic background. Her parents came from Mexico. Consistent with that, family is very important to her.
Instrumental ADL: Care of others: B.B. expresses concern for the well-being of her sister and brothers.		
Child rearing: Student is responsible for all levels of care for her two children, ages 10 and 3. She has selected her mother as a caregiver when B.B. is away.	Beliefs: B.B. adheres to the belief of doing her personal best.	Personal: B.B. is a 31-year-old unemployed nontraditional college student with a high school diploma. She is a former factory worker.
Communication management: Interviewer has observed B.B. communicating on the phone in Spanish with her husband, children, and mother. She communicates clearly in English with non-Spanish-speaking individuals.	Spirituality: B.B. finds meaning in church and a recognition of God. Body functions: Mental: B.B. exhibits sound judgment in driving, problem solving, memory, awareness of reality. She exhibits coping skills when struggles come. She is not known to have any cognitive, affective, or perceptual problems.	Physical: B.B. lives in a ranch house with her husband and two children in a rural area in a subdivision.
Community mobility: B.B. drives where she needs to go and, for exercise, walks to her mother's house in her neighborhood. She also collaborated with a fellow student to arrange carpool plans for her schooling.	Body structures: The student has no known deficiency in body structures.	Social: B.B. does not have a lot of casual friendships. She is close to her husband, mother, and children. She has an adult sister and two grown brothers.
Financial management: B.B. collaborates with her husband regarding their finances.	*Performance Skills* Sensory perceptual skills: B.B. is free of deficiency in this area.	Temporal: B.B. worked for several years in a factory and in an office position. She only recently quit her full-time job to complete her education.
Health management and maintenance: B.B. seems to understand the need for healthy routines. She walks and maintains an active lifestyle with her children. She does not participate in risky behavior.	Motor and praxis skills: The interviewer has observed B.B. performing various motor and praxis skills without difficulty: manipulating keys, driving, maintaining balance while compensating for her book-bag, bending, and reaching.	Virtual: B.B. uses the computer, internet, and cell phone for both calling and texting. *(continued)*

OCCUPATIONS	PERSON	CONTEXT/ENVIRONMENT
Meal preparation and clean-up: B.B. is proactive in planning meals and enjoys finding new recipes to try. She plans and prepares food as well for her Sunday School class. She finds planning parties for family members easy because she has done it many times. Planning and cooking to feed 30 to 50 people is not difficult for her. Religious observance: B.B. is actively involved in her church. B.B. is independent and competent in safety and shopping. Rest and sleep: B.B. does not have any known problems with sleeping. Education: B.B. is a high school graduate. Prior to the present occupational therapy program, she had no college experience. The student is independent and functioning in the program in which she has been enrolled since December. This included 1 year of preparatory general education courses. Work: not applicable Play/leisure: B.B. plays with her children in a variety of activities: hopscotch, jump rope, trampoline, walking, video games. Cooking is not just an instrumental ADL; B.B. enjoys cooking for a hobby as well. Social participation: B.B. engages with her church group, Sunday School children, and family activities, including taking lead roles such as planning meals and activities.	Emotional regulation skills: B.B. is responsive to others' feelings and is quick to express support. She displays emotions appropriate to situations, whether mild or extreme. She persists appropriately despite frustrations. Cognitive skills: The student displays good cognitive skills, such as organizing herself for school, making arrangements and scheduling time to meet for carpooling appointments, and planning her route to school to avoid construction. Communication and social skills: In the classroom setting, B.B. is aware of when to speak and when not to speak. She understands taking turns and acknowledging another people's perspectives. She uses hand gestures to emphasize or describe.	*Performance Patterns* Habits: B.B. does not exhibit any abnormal habits or compulsive behaviors. She automatically locks her car when she leaves it and shows normal safe driving habits. Routines: B.B. displays healthy, organized routines of packing her lunch and organizing her books for school. She organizes herself to leave shortly after school is finished to go home and plans her afternoon by alternating studying and spending time with her kids. Roles: B.B. has a role of mother to two children (elementary age and preschool age). She is a wife and a homemaker. Rituals: Unknown

Reprinted with permission of Lauri Chupp.

Student Sample 6

Sample of Self Occupational Profile

Student Interviewed: K.C.   Date: 9-10-14

This profile is designed to gain an overview of your perspective, occupations, and context/environment, including patterns of daily living, interests, values, and needs. Consult the *OTPF* (AOTA, 2008) for definitions of the terms listed below. You are to summarize significant information for yourself after completing the Activity Configuration.

OCCUPATIONS	PERSON	CONTEXT/ENVIRONMENT
Areas	*Client Factors*	
Activities of daily living (ADL): Shower – flexible; eating and feeding – don't like to cook but enjoy eating; personal hygiene and grooming are important to me	Values: Honesty, fairness, integrity, treat others as I want to be treated, and feel it's important to serve my community	Cultural: Introducing myself, shaking hands, and looking someone in the eyes when speaking
Instrumental ADL: Care of pet	Beliefs: Hard work pays off, important to have work/play balance in life, and one person can make a difference	Personal: 40-year-old female student and administrative assistant
Home management: Single, everything falls on me		Physical: Own home and school facility
Financial management: Important to keep a savings and retirement account	Spirituality: Not religious but do believe in God, we are all a part of each other and nature, I see God in flowers, sunsets, the ocean, etc.	Social: Friends, family members, and colleagues
Shopping: Right now, just shop for needs, not wants	Body functions: Most are okay, would like to work on self-esteem and a better body image; need to work on getting physically fit. Asthma, seasonal allergies, heartburn, and indigestion on occasion	Temporal: Just starting midlife
		Virtual: Use of iPad, smart phone, internet on daily basis, and occasionally a land line
Rest and sleep: Try to rest at times because do not get enough sleep		
Sleep preparation: Lock doors and turn off lights		*Performance Patterns*
Sleep participation: Not as much as I would like, 4 to 6 hours a night	Body structures: Most are okay, lungs (asthma and allergies), some digestive problems (heartburn and indigestion)	Habits: Driving to school, putting car keys and school bag in same place, like to be organized, otherwise feel anxious
Education: Formal education participation: Most important priority in my life right now	*Performance Skills*	
Work: Work as much as needed to just get by; volunteer participation for three different organizations currently	Sensory perceptual skills: All work well for the most part, vision and hearing are not what they used to be; hearing not great when a lot of background noise is present	
	Motor and praxis skills: All work well	

(continued)

OCCUPATIONS	PERSON	CONTEXT/ENVIRONMENT
Play/leisure: Not much time available for this; however, I feel it's important to have in life Social participation: Very important – friends, family, and community	Emotional regulation skills: For the most part are balanced, do not always express feelings to others, working on it and getting better Cognitive skills: All are great and in working order Communication and social skills: Over the years have become much more skilled at this, age and life experience have helped immensely	Routines: Follow same morning sequence of waking up, showering, dressing, and eating and have routine days when I clean out the cat's litter box Roles: Student, friend, sister, aunt, volunteer organization board member and participant Rituals: When reading a book, only stop on even-numbered chapters to mark place until read again; at night, check garage door is closed, doors are locked, and lights are off before can lay down to sleep; buy items that come in multiples like apples or yogurt in even numbers

Reprinted with permission of Kate Campbell.

Student Sample 7

Sample of Self Occupational Profile

Student Interviewed: C.R.   Date: 10-03-14

This profile is designed to gain an overview of your perspective, occupations, and context/environment, including patterns of daily living, interests, values, and needs. Consult the *OTPF* (AOTA, 2008) for definitions of the terms listed below. You are to summarize significant information for yourself after completing the Activity Configuration.

OCCUPATIONS	PERSON	CONTEXT/ENVIRONMENT
Areas Activities of daily living (ADLs): Shower daily in the morning, eat breakfast, lunch, and dinner daily, personal device care—contact lenses and glasses, personal hygiene and grooming—use of razor, deodorant, tweezers, lotions, mousse, make-up, nail polish, hair brush, hair straightener; brush teeth in the morning and before bed Instrumental ADLs: Care of two birds and two daughters; use of cell phone, computer, and iPad; drive a truck for community mobility, bank at a credit union, meal preparation and clean-up daily; grocery shopping weekly Rest and sleep: Rest, 7 to 8 hours of sleep every night; sleep preparation—change into pajamas, brush teeth, tuck girls in, pray, say goodnight, and set alarm clock Education: Pursuing occupational therapy assistant (OTA) degree at Brown Mackie College Work: Currently unemployed, pursuing career as a certified OTA, Student Occupational Therapy Association (SOTA) club participant and treasurer	*Client Factors* Values: Honesty, fairness, commitment to family, and living by the "golden rule" Beliefs: All people are created equal, and hard work pays off Spirituality: We are all God's children, and if we ask, we shall receive Body functions: Emotionally stable, healthy appetite, aware of everything going on around me, decent memory, good hearing, ability to associate taste and smell Body structures: Decent strength and endurance; good eye-hand/foot coordination, all systems of the body functioning normally *Performance Skills* Sensory perceptual skills: Ability to hear and recognize daughters' voices, ability to locate keys in purse, and ability to sense when something is wrong with children Motor and praxis skills: Good coordinating body movements to complete a task, ability to maintain balance adequately, and ability to bend and reach for items	Cultural: Shaking hands when being introduced, kissing on cheek when greeting family members, and respecting elders Personal: 25-year-old woman with two kids who earned GED certificate and is currently working toward degree in occupational therapy Physical: Living in apartment home for over 5 years in Elkhart, Indiana Social: Roles include friend to many, mother to two girls, sister to three brothers, daughter to parents, and student Temporal: Student in the 2-year OTA program at Brown Mackie College Virtual: Use of cell phone, iPad, and Internet daily *Performance Patterns* Habits: Include maintaining a clean environment around me at all times Routines: Include following the same morning sequence to complete showering and grooming in the mornings and cleaning up after every activity

(continued)

OCCUPATIONS	PERSON	CONTEXT/ENVIRONMENT
Play/leisure: Enjoy playing board games, cards, and video games, watching movies, skating, and swimming Social participation: Spending quality time with family and friends is important, involvement in school and SOTA club	Emotional regulation skills: Respond to the feelings of others, able to relax when nervous, ability to control anger, and able to display the appropriate emotions for the situation Cognitive skills: Ability to select items or tools needed for any activity, prioritize activities throughout the day, ability to multitask, organize activities, and sequence tasks to complete a homework assignment Communication and social skills: Ability to acknowledge another person's opinion and recognize facial gestures and body language	Roles: Include mother of a 7-year-old and a 4-year-old, OTA student at Brown Mackie College, and treasurer of SOTA club Rituals: Thank God every morning as soon as I wake up

Reprinted with permission of Cindia Reyes.

Worksheet 2-5

Collage Directions

Construct a collage based on the information you obtained from the person you interviewed.

Collage (pronounced k*uh*-lahzh) is an activity used in occupational therapy for treating a wide variety of conditions with patients/clients throughout the lifespan. The techniques used in creating a collage involve all areas of performance skills listed in the Occupational Therapy Domain. The word *collage* means "to paste," coming from the French word *coller*. Different kinds of paper, with or without images or words, are pasted onto a flat surface to create a symbolic representation of the artist's ideas or impressions. When three dimensional components are included, the collage is called an *assemblage* (Walford, 2002, p. 449).

Use the information gained from your peer to symbolically portray what you know about him or her to create your collage. The following words need to be included in your product:

- Two descriptive words (adjectives)

- Two action words (verbs)

- One phrase (brief statement) that gives your overall impression of this person

- One word that reflects his or her essence from your perspective

  No other words are to appear on the collage.

You are required to use a minimum of 3 media such as photos; three-dimensional objects; and/or crayons, pastels, watercolors, or colored pencils. Be prepared to introduce your peer to the class without revealing his or her name.

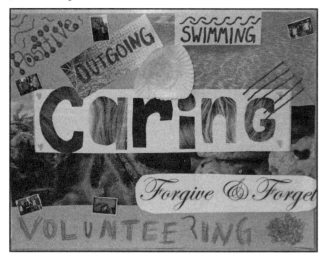

Student Sample 8. Collage. (Reprinted with permission of Stephanie Mareska.)

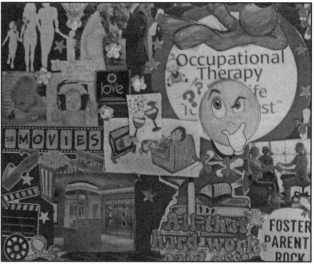

Student Sample 9. Collage. (Reprinted with permission of Kelly Smith.)

Benefits of Creativity: Building Professional Skills
Defining/identifying creativity
Recognizing/acknowledging use of creativity in OT
Describing the cognitive process of creativity
Understanding the neuroscience and structures of creativity
Incorporating creativity into professional skills
Applying creativity in client intervention
Applying research in creativity

3

Relationship of Cognition to Creativity

Marsha Neville, PhD, MS, OT

Creativity is the cognitive process of developing novel and useful solutions to new circumstances. Although creativity may sound like problem solving, a distinction can be made between everyday problem solving and the use of creativity to solve a problem. Creativity is a dynamic process that requires flexibility in approach and thought to develop a practical and effective solution to a novel circumstance. What makes any solution a creative one is the use of an original, out-of-the-ordinary, effective approach to resolve difficulties in a specific situation.

How does one develop creative thinking? Often, people are heard to say "I am not creative." Although perhaps not a painter of great masterpieces or a composer of music, the average person possesses the neuronal structures and the ability to engage in the creative process. Similar to other high levels of cognitive processing, creative thinking involves a complex network of neuronal connections. This network results in the integration of many separate processes working together to express creative responses. Cognitive processes that have been linked to creative thinking include orientation, attention, memory, problem solving, explicit and implicit knowledge, decision making, inhibition of automatic responses, and adaptive behavior in response to novel activities.

This chapter briefly defines the cognitive functions that are linked to creative thinking, discusses current theories of intelligence and its connection to creativity, and details the roles of general knowledge and professional knowledge in thinking creatively. Exercises to illustrate the use of creative thinking are included to help students experience the process involved.

Objectives

1. Identify the cognitive components of creative thinking.

2. Understand how executive functions, coupled with knowledge and intelligence, are thought to produce creative problem solving.

3. Recognize how creative thinking on the part of an occupational therapist changed the approach to and outcome for a client returning home after a hip replacement in a foreign country.

All occupational therapy practitioners possess foundational knowledge of how to plan and provide treatments that serve the client's best interests. The American Occupational Therapy Association (AOTA) provides

Coffey MS, Lamport NK, Hersch GI.
Creative Engagement in Occupation: Building Professional Skills (pp 41-47).
© 2015 SLACK Incorporated.

practice guidelines for treating clients with many medical conditions that require the services of an occupational therapy practitioner, for example, a client with the diagnosis of status post total hip replacement. This is a common diagnosis in adult rehabilitation, and a client with an uncomplicated recovery would benefit from a treatment plan following the AOTA guidelines. However, the client in the case discussed here was not typical, and several unique factors led to a different approach to treating her to help her return home.

Occupational therapy practitioners are often faced with unique problems that demand creative problem solving. Experienced therapists rely on vast amounts of knowledge accumulated in practice and develop an elasticity in thinking to manipulate information to best meet the client's needs. The therapist's knowledge and experience in our example case were used to effectively meet the client's discharge goal. Although she was aware of the AOTA guidelines, the therapist adapted the client's treatment because the treatment demands did not fit those guidelines.

The client lived in England, and while visiting her family in Texas, she broke her hip. The home to which she planned to return was a 300-year-old cottage with cobblestone road access. She had few modern appliances in the kitchen, just a wood-burning stove and a refrigerator. Her bathroom contained an iron tub and no shower. She lived in a small village, and community mobility involved walking to desired locations as an everyday occurrence. For insurance reasons, she was required to return to England. It was clear that this client had an atypical situation and required novel treatment solutions on the part of the therapist. Knowledge of hip precautions and contraindications were indicated for the client, but the therapist also needed to be aware that the client's home, equipment needs, and required modifications were not necessarily the same as those for an individual in her condition being discharged to a home in the United States. In such a situation, the therapist would draw upon multiple sources and use several approaches to resolve typical problems with creative solutions. What cognitive functions are involved in thinking in an out-of-the-ordinary way, and how would the therapist create the solutions needed?

Unit 1: Cognitive Functions

Cognition can be thought of as an umbrella term that encompasses multiple brain functions. Components of cognition include orientation, attention, memory, problem solving, decision making, metacognition, and creativity.

Orientation

Commonly, *orientation* is defined as an awareness of person, place, time, and events (Zoltan, 2007). Such awareness may seem elementary, but orientation is critical for daily function. An awareness of person requires a stored memory of self that includes identifying information (e.g., name or age) and an awareness of all that defines what makes up a person. An awareness of place and recent events requires some storage and processing of surroundings based on perceptual information, prior knowledge, and recent memories. The awareness of time (i.e., date) can be supported by memory, but it can also be aided by the use of clocks, calendars, and environmental cues (e.g., outside sunlight). However, knowing to use aids to determine the date or time requires problem-solving abilities. The awareness of time and date is also supported by routines. A loss of routine can affect any of us. Students often have classes scheduled on Mondays and Wednesdays or Tuesdays and Thursdays. What happens when a Monday holiday causes a change in routine? Students may experience disorientation in preparing for class on Tuesday, packing the wrong books and planning their day based on the Monday schedule. Reorienting oneself requires a conscious effort to override the erroneous sense of time with a corrected version.

Attention

Attention is defined as an effortful, dynamic process that directs our senses to relevant and meaningful events (Zoltan, 2007). There are many different types of attention, including basic arousal, concentration/vigilance, divided attention, and selected attention. Attention responses can be *automatic*, such as turning toward a loud sound, or *intentional*, such as listening to a lecture. Attention can be altered depending on the demand of the task. Overlearned activities, such as walking and driving, are carried out automatically until a person or object intervenes and one is required to change path or speed. In other circumstances, we are aware of the demands for our attention, and we can direct our senses to one stimulus while suppressing competing stimulation (*selected attention*). *Divided attention* is defined as the ability to attend to and switch attention between tasks. Divided attention allows for maintenance of focus on more than one task, although not simultaneously. Tasks and demands may require not only a directing of focus, but also vigilance and sustained attention over a period of time. *Vigilance* can be defined as directed attention that is conscious and lasts for 30 seconds. *Sustained attention*, like vigilance, is conscious directed attention to a task for an extended period of time (Zoltan, 2007, p. 195).

Memory

Memories occur as a result of encoding, storing, and retrieving information. Although a fascinating topic for study, a theoretical discussion of the process of storing and retrieving memories is beyond the scope of this text. Memory involves connections between the brain's hemispheres and between the temporal, parietal, occipital, and frontal lobes. In addition, memories linked to emotions and feelings use networks that engage the amygdala. As with attention, *memory* is a term that encompasses different types of memory. Classically, in neuroscience, terms used to categorize memory include *explicit* and *implicit, declarative* and *nondeclarative, semantic* and *episodic, prospective, procedural, long-term,* and *working/ short-term memory.*

Explicit Memory

Explicit memory is a conscious awareness of how knowledge was obtained. For a memory to be explicit, the person must be able to identify the circumstances surrounding the learning process.

Implicit Memory

Implicit memory is nonconscious knowledge that is used without awareness of the circumstances related to how the knowledge was obtained. Implicit memories include the varied knowledge we have but cannot recall how we obtained it.

Declarative Memory

Declarative memory is a recall of past events and facts. Such events and facts may include episodic memory, declarative memory, and/or semantic memory.

Nondeclarative Memory

Nondeclarative memory is a recall of learned knowledge without awareness of when, where, or how the learning occurred. Nondeclarative memory includes motor skills (e.g., dancing), perceptual skills (e.g., distinguishing a nickel from a dime), and cognitive skills (e.g., knowing to take an umbrella when it is cloudy). A person may see each of these examples as simplistic in how they lack conscious awareness of how the information was learned.

Semantic Memory

Semantic memory involves our memory for general facts and knowledge about ourselves and the world. Semantic memory is relied upon to define who we are and our interests, background, and philosophies. It also involves our vast knowledge of facts about the world, including knowing that summer is hot, that winter is cold, the name of the current president of the United States, and that January 1 starts a new year.

Episodic Memory

Episodic memory involves our memory of the details of personal events. Episodic memories contribute to our recollection of traumatic events along with joyful events. These events can be recalled with great detail, often transporting the person recalling the event to that point in the past.

Prospective Memory

Prospective memory involves remembering future activities and demands and is triggered when we remember to call a friend to check on a meeting time, recall a hair appointment, or remember to bring an assignment to class.

Procedural Memory

Procedural memory refers to our knowledge of how to perform a process or procedure such as riding a bicycle or opening a can. The processes and procedures seem to occur without effort and at a subconscious level. Procedural memories are highly rehearsed activities. It might be said that procedural memory is nondeclarative motor skills.

Long-Term Memory

Long-term memory involves the storage and retrieval of information for future use and requires conscious, effortful rehearsal for consolidation of the content. Long-term memory does not have a storage limit, and information can be retrieved on the basis of the demand of the task.

Working/Short-Term Memory

Working or *short-term memory* entails a conscious, dynamic process of manipulating and filtering information. Information in working memory will not be retained without converting the information to long-term storage, which entails rehearsal with the intent to store information. Working memory is able to manipulate approximately seven pieces of information at one time (depending on how the information is grouped) and is linked to higher intellectual function (Baddeley, 2003).

In summary, cognitive functions include orientation, attention, and memory. As already defined, these cognitive functions entail a vast amount of information processing that includes knowledge of facts, experiences, and skills. In addition, working memory enables us to manipulate approximately seven pieces of information for problem solving and, in some cases, creative problem solving.

Unit 2: Executive Functions

The term *executive function*, like attention or memory, is multidimensional. For purposes of this text, *executive function* will be defined as the overseer of high-order information processing that responds to internal and external demands to perform goal-directed behavior. Executive functions include initiation, directed attention, planning and sequencing, manipulation and retrieval of information, error correction, decision making, flexibility in thinking, and metacognition. Executive functions promote adaptation to new situations and problem solving (Burgess, 1997).

Unit 3: Subprocesses of Executive Function

Planning and Sequencing

Planning and *sequencing* require recognition of a need for action and a breaking down of steps in a methodical, logical sequence. An example of the process is planning a meal. You will need to plan the menu, make the grocery list, buy the groceries, and cook the meal. The meal must be prepared on the correct day and at the correct time.

Manipulating and Retrieving Information

Manipulating and *retrieving information* may sound like using working memory and retrieving stored information, and for our purposes, they can be thought of as the same. Whereas working memory and the retrieval of information are considered forms of memory, their role in executive function is derived from the use of the information to achieve a goal. If we return to the example of planning a dinner, manipulating and retrieving information may include remembering what your guest prefers to eat, what you have cooked in the past, and where you have stored needed recipes.

Problem Solving/Decision Making

Problem solving and *decision making* may be thought of as connected forms of processing. They both require conscious attention to the manipulation of options to achieve a goal. In the example of planning a meal, you learn that your guest has a newly discovered peanut allergy, but you had planned a Thai dinner that included peanut sauce. Your executive function system recognizes the problem, and you must decide on a solution. This shift in the plan requires that you use flexible thinking.

Flexible Thinking

Flexible thinking involves the ability to shift gears and scrap or modify a plan. To avoid a disastrous dinner, you will need to change the items on the menu or modify your recipe.

Metacognition

Metacognition is one's ability to understand oneself, a self-awareness of strengths, weaknesses, and capabilities. Using metacognition, you as a meal planner know that you are good at making stir-fry recipes, but you can also make other dishes. You have a sense of what skills and abilities you possess that will enable you to achieve your goal of preparing the meal.

Unit 4: Knowledge and Intelligence

As with all definitions of the constructs of cognitive function and executive function, the fields of neuroscience, psychology, education, and data management have sought to explain the process of knowledge and intelligence. For the purposes of this text, I will present more generic and broad definitions.

Knowledge

Knowledge can be defined as knowing facts, truths, principles, and skills. It can be explicit (the person has an awareness of when and how he or she learned the information) or implicit (the person knows the information without a conscious awareness of how, when, or where he or she obtained it). Knowledge is often used synonymously with the term *information*, but it could be argued that information may or may not be valid and reliable. Knowledge, on the other hand, is argued to have evidence and support for its reliability and validity. One might read information in a gossip magazine, but it may not be equal to knowledge (facts, truths, and principles). Knowledge can be validated by credible sources and outcomes when related to skill (Alexander, Winters, Loughlin, & Grossnickle, 2012).

Intelligence

When defining intelligence, as when defining other facets of cognition, the intelligent person must understand that it is not absolute. Our understanding of the brain and its complexity is a vast field of unknowns and not totally understood. It would be a mistake to say that we understand the complex mechanisms of thought, learning, knowledge, and information manipulation. That said, *intelligence* has been defined as the ability to reason, problem solve, critically think, make abstractions, and understand complex issues. Individuals differ in intelligence performance depending on their experiences and knowledge and how they adapt and learn from their experiences. An individual's intelligence can also differ depending on the demands and domain. Davis, Christodoulou, Seider, and Gardner (2011) proposed that intelligence is multidimensional and identified the following eight domains of intelligence: spatial, linguistic, logical-mathematical, bodily-kinesthetic, musical, interpersonal, intrapersonal, and naturalistic.

In the original Triarchic Theory of Intelligence and, more recently, the Theory of Successful Intelligence, Sternberg (1985, 2003) proposed that the three facets of intelligence are analytic intelligence, creative intelligence, and practical intelligence. *Analytic intelligence* is defined as the mental process (e.g., critical thinking, problem solving, and abstracting). *Creative intelligence* is used when a person is confronted with a novel problem or situation. *Practical intelligence* is bound by societal rules and principles, pragmatics of the context, and environmental constraints.

UNIT 5: CREATIVITY

Understanding the components of cognitive functions and information processing provides some foundation for understanding creativity. There are a number of theoretical models that attempt to describe and define creativity, and the study of creativity is a growing field in neuroscience. The focus of this discussion involves creativity as it relates to problem solving and critical thinking. Other areas of study examine creativity in the context of artistic expression, which is beyond the scope of this chapter. A broad and inclusive definition of *creativity* would be the ability to develop original and valuable solutions in a given situation. Original solutions can include new, unique, or unexpected ideas or actions. A solution is considered valuable when it is useful, appropriate, practical, or adaptive. Most researchers would support the idea that for a solution to be creative, it must be both original and valuable (Dietrich, 2004b; Fink, Benedek, Grabner, Staudt, & Neubauer, 2007).

Creativity is a multifaceted, complex form of information processing. In general, all components of cognitive function and executive function contribute to creative problem solving. The brain consists of a complex network of highways connecting multiple areas and contributing to multiple pathways. Creativity, along with other cognitive functions, benefits from these highways. Many, if not all, of the cognitive and executive functions outlined here are thought to contribute to creativity. Thinking of creativity as a construct, we might believe that the cognitive and executive functions of self-awareness, attention (both focused and defocused), memory (working, long term, explicit, implicit, procedural, and declarative), and planning and initiation play roles in creative thinking. Other terms used to describe the components of creativity are *insightful thinking*, *divergent thinking*, *ideational fluency* (generating ideas), *novelty* (uniqueness and originality), and *flexibility of mind* (variation of ideas) (Fink et al., 2007). Dietrich (2004a, 2007) argued that creative thinking requires working memory, sustained attention, and cognitive flexibility. How knowledge and intelligence support creativity is a growing field of research. Knowledge and intelligence are stored in memory and provide support for creative thinking, and depending on experiences and areas of study, the levels of knowledge and intelligence a person possesses may influence his or her level of creative thinking. In other words, a person might be creative in solving complex math problems but not in the area of environmental adaptations. Creativity also requires knowledge of rules and pragmatics, and environmental, cultural, and social confounds must be considered. What might be a novel, effective solution in one context or culture may not be so in another context, culture, or society (Carlsson, Wendt, & Risberg, 2000; Dietrich, 2004b).

UNIT 6: FROM COGNITION TO CREATIVITY

In this chapter, the components of cognition, executive functions, knowledge, intelligence, and creativity have been explained. Daily use of cognitive skills for activities such as maintaining a schedule, learning, remembering an appointment, planning for future events, anticipating needs, recognizing danger, and adapting to change and near-unconscious performance of motor tasks such as walking, driving, and dressing often occur with little more than an afterthought. Yet, each of these activities requires some level of self-awareness, attention, memory, knowledge, and intelligence. The process of creativity within the context of cognitive function seems to demand additional resources that cause a person to stop, think, manipulate, manipulate some more, weigh choices, and develop a solution. Unlike daily problem solving, creativity requires a person to solve a novel or unique problem with a practical and/or productive outcome that is suitable to the context, culture, and society in which the person resides.

Let's revisit the client who is returning to England after a hip replacement. She will need to adhere to hip precautions that prohibit her from flexing her hip more than 90 degrees or rotating her hip. Although some occupational therapy guidelines can meet the client's needs (e.g., reacher and long-handled sponge), the client's standard toilet is European and higher than American toilets. Through adaptation of the bathroom and practice, the patient is able to perform safe transfers. Two major deterrents to the patient's progress are using the tub and community mobility. The therapist knows that the patient will need a method of bathing that does not require her to lower herself into the tub. She questions the use of a plank across the tub (marble or stone). She proposes trying it to determine the practicality of such an adaptation. To help with rinsing, hoses that can be adapted to the faucet were explored. It might be argued that these adaptations required minimal creativity, and that might be so. In addition to these solutions, the therapist built a simulated cobblestone path with paver tiles at the hospital for practice. Although a standard walker was difficult to manipulate, the patient reported access to a battery-operated scooter that she could use to get to town. In practice, she also discovered that certain shoes were better for walking on the stones and that a four-pronged cane vs a straight cane was best for her.

To enhance your awareness of the components of creative thinking, a number of exercises have been included. These exercises may be completed individually or in small groups. During participation in the exercise, you are encouraged to think about the thought processes required to perform the exercise. Again, note that no component of cognition is used in isolation. For every exercise or activity, a number of components will be used.

Activity 3-1: Combining Ideas

Exercise 3-1A

Step 1: Define and explain each of the following words using as many descriptors and definitions as you can think of: apple, hammer.

Step 2: Now combine the two words to develop ideas on how they relate to each other or could be used together.

Exercise 3-1B

Step 1: Define and explain each of the following words using as many descriptors and definitions as you can think of: tractor, harp.

Step 2: Now combine the two words to develop ideas on how they relate to each other or could be used together.

Activity 3-2: Metacognition

Instructions: Answer the following questions using reflective thinking. *Reflective thinking* may best be defined as "thinking about your thinking."

1. What have you learned about cognition? Provide a reflection of how this has impacted your knowledge for future use.
2. What have you learned about executive function? Provide a reflection of how it has affected your knowledge.
3. Explain creativity; include some reflection on the subcomponents.
4. Give an example of a time in your past when you believe you used creative problem solving, and discuss the cognitive processing that you recall using.

Grading

- 3 points: Demonstrates reflective thinking at a depth of understanding that relies on more than the information provided in this chapter; draws from other information.
- 2 points: Some reflective thinking but lacks depth and reflective understanding from past experience.
- 1 point: Answered questions with little reflection of thought processes and knowledge; reflected rephrasing of information.

Conclusion

As in everyday life, therapy can often be routine and follow standard guidelines. However, when circumstances require novel and practical solutions, the therapist can use creative problem solving. The therapist is required to recognize the incongruence in standard treatment and the needs of the client; attend to pertinent details; have knowledge of equipment and compare present to past experiences; imagine novel, never-seen environments; and consider myriad possible solutions.

Questions

1. After completing the exercise, what components of cognition can you identify as having performed yourself? Compare your experience with that of a peer.

2. Has your awareness of your own creativity changed by completing an exercise? If so, which exercise produced this awareness, and did the experience confirm or negate your ability to be creative?

3. What application can this type of exercise have for a friend? An occupational therapy practitioner? A client?

References

Alexander, P., Winters, F., Loughlin, S., & Grossnickle, E. (2012). Students' conceptions of knowledge, information, and truth. *Learning & Instruction, 22*(1), 1-15.

Baddeley, A. (2003). Working memory: looking back and looking forward. *Nature Reviews: Neuroscience, 4*(10), 829-839.

Burgess, P. W. (1997). *Theory and methodology in executive function research, in methodology of frontal and executive function* (ed. P. Rabbitt). New York, NY: Psychology Press, pp. 81-166.

Carlsson, I., Wendt, P., & Risberg, J. (2000). On the neurobiology of creativity: Differences in frontal activity between high and low creative subjects. *Neuropsychologia, 38*(6), 873-885.

Davis, K., Christodoulou, J., Seider, S., & Gardner, H. (2011). The theory of multiple intelligences. In R. Sternberg, & S. B. Kaufman, S. B. (Eds.), *The Cambridge handbook of intelligence* (pp. 485-503). New York, NY: Cambridge University Press.

Dietrich, A. (2004a). Neurocognitive mechanisms underlying the experience of flow. *Consciousness and Cognition, 13*(4), 746-761.

Dietrich, A. (2004b). The cognitive neuroscience of creativity. *Psychonomic Bulletin & Review, 11*(6), 1011-1026.

Dietrich, A. (2007). Who's afraid of a cognitive neuroscience of creativity? *Methods, 42*(1), 22-27.

Fink, A., Benedek, M., Grabner, R., Staudt, B., & Neubauer, A. (2007). Creativity meets neuroscience: Experimental tasks for the neuroscientific study of creative thinking. *Methods, 42*(1), 68-76.

Sternberg, R. J. (1985). *Beyond IQ: A triarchic theory of human intelligence.* New York, NY: Cambridge University Press.

Sternberg, R. J. (2003). A broad view of intelligence: The theory of successful intelligence. *Consulting Psychology Journal: Practice & Research, 55*(3), 139-154.

Zoltan, B. (2007). *Vision, perception, and cognition: A manual for the evaluation and treatment of the adult with acquired brain injury* (4th ed.). Thorofare, NJ: SLACK, Incorporated.

Benefits of Creativity:
Building Professional Skills

Defining/identifying creativity

Recognizing/acknowledging use of creativity in OT

Describing the cognitive process of creativity

Understanding the neuroscience and structures of creativity

Incorporating creativity into professional skills

Applying creativity in client intervention

Applying research in creativity

4

Neurological Implications of Creativity

Mary Frances Baxter, PhD, LOT, FAOTA

Until recently, the study of creativity and the study of neuroscience were considered mutually exclusive, requiring different mechanisms and theories for acquiring knowledge. Now, understanding creativity from a neuroscience perspective is a growing field, as evidenced by the results of bringing the two disciplines together through a common body of literature (Abraham & Windman, 2007; Dietrich, 2007). Technologies developed in the past 20 years, including magnetic resonance imaging, functional magnetic resonance imaging, and positron emission tomography, are used in the neurosciences to study brain functions (Fink, Benedek, Grabner, Staudt, & Neubauer, 2007; Fink et al., 2009; Jung et al., 2009; Mölle et al., 1996). These technologies are helping to provide an understanding of the creative processes that occur in the brain. In addition, studies completed with persons identified with abnormal brain function and progressive neurological diseases are opening windows to our comprehension of creativity (Bogousslavsky, 2005; Cummings, Miller, Christensen, & Cherry, 2008; Miller, Ponton, Benson, Cummings, & Mena, 1996).

This chapter is not meant to provide a foundation on brain structures and functions but is written to provide an understanding of creativity from a neuroscience perspective. This information gives us a basis for examining the potential of individuals to be creative, whether one is a student, a therapist, or a client. It provides us with incentive to explore options and unexpected solutions in occupational therapy treatment methods and outcomes.

OBJECTIVES

1. Identify the structures of the central nervous system (CNS) involved in creativity.

2. Discover how neurotransmitters and the transmission of information in the CNS contribute to creativity.

3. Describe how the processes taking place in those with mental illness and in those who are aging have contributed to our understanding of creativity.

4. Summarize how, from a neuroscience perspective, the creative process contributes to one's health.

There are many definitions of creativity and a variety of models for uncovering and understanding the mechanisms that produce creativity. A generally accepted model of creativity, originally proposed by Wallas in 1926, involves examining creative output through the following four-stage process: preparation, incubation,

Coffey MS, Lamport NK, Hersch GI.
Creative Engagement in Occupation: Building Professional Skills (pp 49-59).
© 2015 SLACK Incorporated.

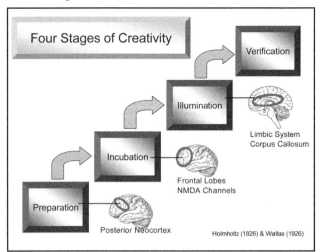

Figure 4-1. Stages of creativity.

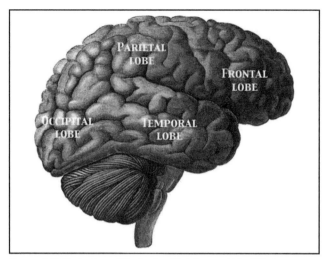

Figure 4-2. Illustration of the brain with lobes and identified areas.

illumination, and verification (Heilman, 2005; Wallas, 1926) (Figure 4-1). *Preparation* is development of the knowledge and skills required to do a task, which includes a basic predisposition or talent for performing that task; it also requires understanding, training, and experience for creative output. *Incubation* is a period of time when notions, ideas, and directed thinking are set aside. Moments of insight come during a temporary distraction or relaxation. Ramon y Cajal (1852-1934), a father of modern neuroscience, lends credence to the need for incubation. In his book *Advice for a Young Investigator*, he wrote "If a solution fails to appear…and yet we feel success is just around the corner, try resting for a while. Several weeks of relaxation and quiet in the countryside bring calmness and clarity of the mind" (Cajal, 1916, p. 35). *Illumination* is the "aha!" moment, that moment when an undiscovered thought or idea is revealed, often after a period of incubation. Finally, the output of the creative process requires *verification* to justify the idea or completed work as a result of using the "new" approach. This verification may come from the scientific community, mathematics, or another source. Verification also may occur through the confirmation or affirmation of those who apply the creative output that resulted from the process.

Each of these four stages of creativity may be traced to different structures in the brain (Figure 4-2).

UNIT 1: STRUCTURES AND FUNCTIONS OF THE CENTRAL NERVOUS SYSTEM: A BRIEF OVERVIEW

Roles of the Central Nervous System in Creativity

Cognition is the term used to describe a wide range of tasks processed by the brain. Simple cognitive processes include tasks such as seeing, hearing, and responding to pain or fear. At the more complex end of the spectrum are the higher cognitive functions, known as *executive functions*. These include attention, perception, memory, insight, and abstract thinking. Creativity is also considered a higher cognitive function by most neuroscientists who study it. The neural basis for the higher cognitive functions is the cerebral cortex of the brain. Recent theories of the neural correlates of cognition put emphasis on the frontal cortex for providing these higher attributes, including self-awareness, problem solving, divergent thinking, and other executive functions. Research also suggests that the entire brain can be activated when people are engaged in creative tasks (Fink et al., 2009; Heilman, Nadeau, & Beversdorf, 2003). Furthermore, it is well established that neuronal activity patterns in the cerebral cortex change in response to lived experiences and learning (Buonomano & Merzenich, 1998; LeDoux, 2002). The postulate is that creativity occurs when preparation through experience and learning takes place, and this is a requirement, not an option.

The preparation stage of creativity is the learning phase, which occurs as areas of knowledge and talent are developed. For instance, painters learn to use tools and paints in particular ways, scientists learn foundational knowledge and learn about techniques used in scientific research, and dancers learn basic movements and steps that provide a foundation for more complex movements. These areas of knowledge and skill development are known as *domain-specific knowledge*. Many researchers in creativity have indicated that domain-specific knowledge is a prerequisite for creativity (Chakravarty, 2010; Dietrich, 2004). Domain-specific knowledge is generally believed to be stored in the posterior neocortex and the posterior temporal lobe. Results of research performed on lesions in the posterior neocortex (posterior frontal lobe) and the posterior temporal lobe indicate that these areas are important in processing and mediating higher cognitive functions, including spatial relations, computation, literacy, and mathematics.

Specific Roles of the Frontal Lobes

Although the brain's frontal lobe is identified as the seat of the highest cognitive functions, it does not receive direct sensory information from the environment as do the temporal, parietal, and occipital lobes. Rather, it integrates information from the other three lobes to enable advanced and complex cognitive behaviors. Research shows that there is an increase in blood flow and neural activity in the frontal lobes, specifically the prefrontal cortex, when creativity takes place (Kalbfleisch, 2004; Mihov, Denzler, & Förster, 2010; Razoumnikova, 2000).

The prefrontal cortex is responsible for working memory, temporal integration, and sustained and directed attention, which provide an infrastructure for processing these cognitive functions. One executive function is *cognitive flexibility*, an ability to see different aspects of an object, idea, or situation while switching attention as needed in the process. Picturing an object from a different angle, attending to multiple tasks while cooking a meal, and imagining a different outcome with changes in a scenario are some examples of seeing different aspects of a situation. Each of these complex mental tasks, used in combination with other cognitive functions, contributes significantly to cognitive flexibility. However, the prefrontal cortex is not a single unit but two functionally divided portions. One part is the *ventromedial prefrontal cortex*, which is connected to the emotional centers of the amygdala and cingulated cortex, suggesting more of a role in social and emotional behaviors. The other part, the *dorsolateral prefrontal cortex*, is connected with the sensory processing centers of the occipital, temporal, and parietal lobes, suggesting a role in the integration of sensory information. Studies have shown that the prefrontal cortices have both an organizing role for integrating information and an inhibitory role for emotional and cognitive functions.

The posterior neocortices sit just behind the frontal cortices. The posterior neocortex functions in processing learning and memory, and there are strong implications that it also is involved in the development of knowledge and skills. This forms a foundation for the preparation phase of creativity to take place, as noted earlier. However, for creativity to be exercised, suppression of cognitive processes of the posterior neocortical regions also needs to occur (Kowatari et al., 2009). This need for the suppression of memory and knowledge suggests that the creative process requires application of memory, knowledge, and skills in new ways, not simply a repeating of what is known or remembered.

Hemispheric Specialization

For a long time, we have used the specialization of the right and left hemispheres of the brain as the basis for understanding creativity. A commonly held belief has been that people who are left-hand dominant are more creative than people who are right-handed. Because the right hemisphere controls the motor functions of the left upper extremity, creativity has been attributed to this side of the brain. Other functions usually associated with the right hemisphere include language capacity and performance, the processing of visual and auditory stimuli, spatial manipulation, facial perception, and artistic ability. In contrast, the left hemisphere is associated with linear reasoning, language functions such as grammar and vocabulary, and numerical manipulation. Because the left hemisphere controls motor functions of the right side of the body, people who are right-handed were considered to have left hemisphere dominance (Kowatari et al., 2009; Mihov et al., 2010).

There is some evidence that well-known visual artists such as Leonardo da Vinci, Michelangelo, and Raphael were left-handed, although there are many visual artists who are right-hand dominant. However, processes besides visual artistry are involved in the expression of creativity, and one notable example is Albert Einstein, who appeared to be right-handed. We now know that hand dominance is not a clear indication of the location of brain function. Using language as an example, the majority (95%) of persons who are right-hand dominant primarily use the left hemisphere for processing language. Yet, only 18.8% of left-handed people have right-hemisphere dominance for language function. Furthermore, 19.8% of those who are left-hand dominant have language functions processed in both hemispheres (Heilman et al., 2003; Taylor & Taylor, 1990).

Recently, researchers using brain-imaging studies have attempted to determine whether creativity is localized in one hemisphere (Heilman et al., 2003; Katz, 1979). The difficulty in performing an analysis of this sort is the variability of the measurements and methodological techniques and of the conceptual foundations for characterizing creativity. Mihov et al. (2010) provided a comprehensive meta-analysis of literature related to creativity and hemispheric specialization. They concluded that "the probability of right hemisphere activation during a creative task is greater than the probability of left hemisphere activation" (p. 444). However, they cautioned that the subprocesses of creativity, such as problem formation, processing, and incubation, were not identified in the literature, only the specific moment of the outcome of the creative process. In addition, the literature they reviewed did not delve into specific brain regions, only lateralization within the brain as a whole.

The results of several more recent studies indicate that creativity requires the activation of regions in both hemispheres along with multiple and divergent brain processes (Kowatari et al., 2009). For instance, writing requires verbal and visual processing of language, but it also requires mental or visual processing of the scenes, actions, or movements that are being described.

Limbic System

The primary roles of the limbic system are to process and mediate emotions and to act as a major contributor in the formation of memories. The structures of the limbic system include the amygdala, the hypothalamus, the hippocampus, and several areas of the cortex, and it is interconnected to many, if not all, parts of the brain. As a result of this interconnectedness, the limbic system is integrated with the sensory systems and provides the mechanisms for processing emotions related to sensations. The limbic system also connects with the autonomic nervous system (ANS) through the hypothalamus and provides the mechanism for the physical responses that occur with stimulation to the ANS, such as the common fight-or-flight response. In addition, the limbic system works with the ventromedial prefrontal cortex to produce and evaluate complex emotional and social situations. Although the limbic system has not been studied extensively as it relates to creativity, its interconnectedness with other CNS systems and its major roles in attention, emotions, learning, and memory make it a significant contributor to and benefactor of creative processes.

Unit 2: Neuroprocessing and Neurotransmission

Neurotransmitters: An Overview

The human body functions and processes information in the CNS via a complicated system comprising nerve cells called *neurons* and chemical messengers called *neurotransmitters*. Neurons are the basic unit for all functions and processes in living beings, from the simple eating patterns of *Aplysia* to the complicated operations of thinking and feeling experienced by humans (Baxter & Byrne, 2006). In the human body, neurons do not touch other nerve cells, but they convey information through nerve pathways to the brain and spinal cord via electrical impulses moving in one direction. The space between neurons in which neurotransmitters circulate is called a *synapse*. The role of the neurotransmitters is to relay signals across the synapse from each neuron to a target cell, often another neuron.

The number of known neurotransmitter types is well over 100. With this many different neurotransmitters, categorization is difficult and has resulted in the use of several systems. A commonly accepted form categorizes them according to their basic chemical structure: 1, the amino acids; 2, the monoamines; and 3, the neuropeptides. A fourth substance, acetylcholine, is often classified in a separate category because it does not fit into any of the other groups and it can be designated as a neurotransmitter type of its own.

The *amino acids* are the most abundant neurotransmitters in the CNS and include glutamate, gamma-aminobutyric acid (GABA), and glycine. Of the amino acid neurotransmitters, glutamate has a major excitatory role and is distributed throughout the brain. GABA is the major inhibitory neurotransmitter in the brain. Our nervous system is designed to be active, but neurons would be overactive and not well controlled without the inhibitory effects of GABA and other neurotransmitters. Inhibition is required so that proper function may occur.

The *monoamines* include neurotransmitters such as dopamine, norepinephrine, epinephrine (adrenaline), and serotonin. These neurotransmitters work in many parts of the CNS and ANS, contributing to wake and sleep cycles, stages of alertness, emotional reactions, stress-level regulation, and the fight-or-flight response. They are also found in many parts of the brain that contribute to learning and memory, including the prefrontal cortex. Chermahini & Hommel (2010) found a correlation between dopamine and creativity, yet also state that the relationship is complex and that the functioning of dopamine relates in different ways to the many varied aspects of creativity. *Norepinephrine* is connected to the retrieval of long-term memory. During tasks that require creative thinking, the amount of this monoamine is reduced. It is surmised that the reduction of norepinephrine in the process of creative thinking helps the brain ignore or forget information stored in memory, thereby allowing novel connections and new ideas to emerge.

Serotonin contributes to mood stability and emotional response. Specifically, serotonin helps the body maintain a feeling of calmness. Conversely, *cortisol* is a hormone that is produced under periods of stress, anxiety, or frustration. Among other detrimental effects, excess cortisol has been shown to inhibit focus, slow the thinking process, and add to depression. Serotonin and cortisol work in opposition to each other to maintain a homeostatic balance within the body. Thus, although not proven, it seems appropriate to suggest that creative processes are best achieved when one's serotonin level is high and the cortisol level is relatively low. To further support this idea, higher levels of serotonin have been found when one is in a state of flow, as described by Mihaly Csikszentmihalyi (1997). *Flow* is defined as a mental state experienced by a person fully immersed in an activity, intentionally focused on the process, and successfully completing a task (Csikszentmihalyi, 1997). Conversely, engaging in creative activities has been shown to reduce cortisol levels, thereby increasing serotonin levels. Elevation of the serotonin level helps a person to increase attention and focus, clarify thinking, and reduce anxiety and stress.

The class of neurotransmitters known as *peptides* includes β-endorphin and other peptide-based neurotransmitters. β-endorphin interacts specifically with opioid receptors in the CNS, promoting a sense of well-being and inducing analgesic responses to pain. The results of some research indicate that the creative process can release endorphins and thereby promote calmness. The release of endorphins through the creative process may also provide a reduction in pain.

Acetylcholine is a neurotransmitter found in all three divisions of the nervous system—the CNS, the ANS, and the peripheral nervous system. In the CNS, acetylcholine plays a role in changing the connection between neurons, specifically how much and how often the neurons interact with each other. This ability of the neurons to change connections is known as *synaptic plasticity*. Synaptic plasticity is critical for learning and building memory; therefore, acetylcholine plays an important role in the preparation phase of creativity. Acetylcholine also has a major role in processing and integrating sensory information. In the peripheral nervous system, acetylcholine mediates sensation and voluntary movement. Lastly, acetylcholine is the primary neurotransmitter in the ANS, regulating cardiac and respiratory muscles. As stated earlier, learning and memory are major contributors to the creative process. Processing sensory information is also critical in creativity. ANS responses, such as fight or flight, are not conducive to creativity. Thus, acetylcholine plays a major role in the creative process through its function in the nervous systems. Furthermore, imbalances in acetylcholine have been found in people with depression and in those with Alzheimer's disease; both of these conditions are known for decreased divergent thinking and a reduction in other forms of creativity.

In review, neurotransmitters are the message carriers for the nervous system and are the basis for essential information processing to take place. They are potentially detrimental and/or enabling in the creative process. It is important to be aware of the detrimental effects of stress (e.g., frustration, fatigue, or pain) on a person's body and on his or her ability to create. At the same time, understanding the beneficial effects of creativity (e.g., reducing stress, frustration, fatigue, or pain) can foster creative client-centered therapy.

UNIT 3: NEUROLOGICAL DISORDERS

Much of what is known about neuroscience and creativity has come from the study of persons with psychosocial and cognitive impairments. There are numerous stories about persons who are identified as highly creative and also exhibit odd behaviors. The painter Vincent Van Gogh was known to have long bouts of depression. Another painter, Salvador Dali, had an affinity for making dangerous animals his pets. Albert Einstein is often cited as one of the most creative men, yet he was known to get tobacco for his pipe from discarded cigarette and cigar remains. Howard Hughes had an unnatural aversion to germs and created germ-free zones in his environment. More recently, vocal artist Michael Jackson had a preoccupation with undergoing plastic surgery. There are many instances in which eccentric behavior and creative output are traits found in the same person. The following is a brief discussion of the neurological basis for creativity in several forms of mental illness and degenerative diseases.

Neurological Disorders and Creativity

Belief in a link between the expression of creativity and mental health disorders has long been held. Indeed, there is much anecdotal evidence for a relationship between creativity and psychosis, particularly schizophrenia. Persons with psychoses are believed to have a capacity to see the world in novel ways, leading to creative outputs. One explanation for the novel thinking and increased creativity associated with people with mental illness is their openness to incoming stimuli from the surrounding environment; this is referred to as *low latent inhibition*. Latent inhibition is defined as the ability to block out or ignore stimuli that are irrelevant to the current situation or needs. Both creative individuals and persons with some mental illnesses have low levels of latent inhibition. Psychologists indicate that it is likely that low levels of latent inhibition and cognitive flexibility may predispose individuals to mental illness under some conditions and to creative accomplishments under others. Neuroscientists indicate that the sensory processing mechanism in the thalamus, the receiver of all sensory stimuli in the human body, is similarly different in highly creative persons and in some persons with mental illness, thus providing a neurological explanation for low levels of latent inhibition (Bogousslavsky, 2005; Cummings et al., 2008; Sellal & Musacchio, 2008).

Other mental illnesses with which creative people are often associated are two of the diagnostic types of bipolar disorder. Bipolar I disorder manifests with severe episodes of mania and depression interspersed with periods of wellness. An increase in the severity of manic episodes can disable a person to the point of being unable to express, in a functional way, the exaggerated perceptions, thoughts, and ideas he or she encounters. Persons with bipolar II disorder experience milder periods of increased mania. During these periods, the randomness of ideas, faster thought processes, and the ability to take in more information can be harnessed for use in creative endeavors. The depressive end of the disorder, however, seems to inhibit creative processes.

Research into the progression of several degenerative diseases has also contributed to an understanding of the neurological basis for creativity. Specifically, there are several case studies of persons with frontotemporal lobar disease (FTLD) that have provided knowledge about the creative process. FTLD is a condition in which the frontal and anterior temporal lobes of the cortex progressively deteriorate. In reports of persons with FTLD, an emergence of creativity, especially in visual art, music, mathematics, and mechanics, has been shown to occur as the disease progresses. This emergence is found in persons who previously had no interest or skill in these areas. This progression of the disease supports the concept, presented earlier, that the suppression of the frontal cortex provides a conduit through which creativity can occur. As the frontal and temporal lobes deteriorate, activity in these areas is reduced, allowing creativity from other cortical areas to emerge. Unfortunately for those with FTLD, the disease continues to progress, and creativity deteriorates along with the other cortical functions (Cummings et al., 2008; Liu et al., 2009; Miller et al., 1996).

Effect of Creativity on Neurological Disorders

Evidence related to the effect of creativity on mental health is inconclusive, but creativity seems to have a protective, even curative effect for those experiencing mental illness. Self-expression, relaxation, decreased blood pressure, and stress reduction are some of the documented benefits of engagement in creative endeavors (Chatterjee, 2004; Daykin, McClean, & Bunt, 2007; Khasky & Smith, 1999). The growing knowledge base, although not yet strong, supports the potential for using creativity as a therapeutic tool and not simply a beneficial diversion.

Unit 4: Aging

Neurological Changes as a Result of Aging

With age, the brain undergoes changes just as the rest of the body does. Specifically, there is an overall loss of neurons, which results in changes to brain morphology. An obvious result is the decreased weight and volume of the brain. Coinciding with these changes is a reduction in the size of many areas of the cerebral cortex. As neurons are depleted and cortical areas are reduced, there is a subsequent enlargement of the ventricles. The *ventricles* are the spaces within the brain that hold and process the cerebrospinal fluid. Another feature of the aging brain is a change in the surface of the brain's hills (*gyri*) and valleys (*sulci*). There is a widening of the sulci, which reduces the overall surface area. As a result of all of these changes, the conditions typically seen in older persons that affect the CNS include Alzheimer's disease, Parkinson's disease, and cerebral vascular accidents (Kim, Hasher, & Zacks, 2008; Kulisevsky, Pagonabarraga, & Martinez-Corral, 2009).

Regardless, there is much information to suggest that the aging brain and the creative brain share similar characteristics. The aging brain is more distractible than its younger counterpart. Psychologist Dr. Lynn Hasher and her colleagues confirmed this increased distractibility in a study comparing attention in older and younger participants (Kim et al., 2008). This, and other research regarding the effects of aging on cognition, suggests that there is a broadening of the focus of attention in the aging brain. In studies of highly creative individuals, this same broadening of attention is indicated. In the study conducted by Hasher, participants in the older group were better able to use the distracting information to solve problems presented later in the study. Using distracting information and combining unrelated information is a characteristic of creativity. Therefore, the widened attention in the aging brain allows an individual to hold and use disparate information in much the same way that a creative person can.

Another characteristic of the aging brain is a lessening of inhibition. As noted earlier, there are reductions in size of many parts of the brain as a result of aging. In particular, the prefrontal cortex, which is involved in self-regulation, self-conscious awareness, and emotions, is an area that is reduced. As a result of this reduction in size, there seems to be a diminished need for an aging person to please and impress others. This characteristic is also present in creative persons. The similarity in older individuals and creative persons is a likelihood of disregarding social conventions and a willingness to speak their minds when compared with their younger counterparts.

Lastly, it is important to present the concept of *crystallized intelligence* and its role in creativity. Crystallized intelligence is the knowledge, skills, and experiences that are gained over a lifetime and the ability of a person to subsequently use them in novel ways. Studies of intelligence with the aging population indicate that older individuals have an increased store of knowledge gained over years of experience and learning. Specifically, on tests of crystallized intelligence, aging brains score better than their younger counterparts, showing an increased store of information. We now know that creativity by definition is the result of using knowledge from different sources and combining information into original ideas. In the creative process, crystallized intelligence is the foundation used to make novel and original associations. Therefore, the aging brain, with its increased bank of knowledge, provides a rich foundation for creative activity and suggests that the elderly are ideally suited for creative endeavors. Productive aging for elders can result from transitioning into cultural activities such as art and music, voluntary participation in community service, and pursuing a second career as an alternative to inactive retirement.

Effect of Creative Endeavors on an Aging Brain

Engagement in learning, building memory, and creative activities helps build more and stronger connections between the neurons in the CNS. This increase in the number of neural connections contributes to cognitive reserve. *Cognitive reserve* is the mind's ability to resist damage to the brain. Thus, even as the brain is losing neurons and size, the behaviors seen as measures of the mind are more resilient. Indeed, much has been written to indicate that the development of cognitive reserve protects the aging person against cognitive decline as well as the effects of dementia. In addition, engagement in creative activities contributes to the growth of such cognitive reserve. Most of the work done on cognitive reserve shows that extended periods or lifetimes of enriched environments and cognitive stimulation provide the protection of cognitive reserve. Yet, researchers Noice, Noice, and Staines (2004) suggest that even a short period in an enriched environment can have positive effects in controlling or reducing cognitive decline by building and maintaining neuronal connectivity in the brain.

The implications of this information are two-fold. First, engaging in a lifetime of creative activities or even in shorter periods of creative activities has the beneficial effects of building cognitive reserve and reducing the potential effects of dementia or other conditions on the brain and cognition. Furthermore, using creative activities in occupational practice can have positive effects on patients who are experiencing cognitive decline.

CONCLUSION

This chapter has presented how creativity is defined and understood from a neuroscience perspective, providing a greater appreciation for the complexity of creativity. In addition, insights have been provided regarding how creativity can change the nervous system, from modulating neurotransmitters to changing the interactions of neurons in different parts of the CNS. The research being done on creativity in neuroscience and in other scientific fields is providing an understanding of creative processes and evidence for using creative activities with persons who receive occupational therapy treatment. By providing purposeful activities that promote problem solving and enhance the potential for the client to draw from his or her inner resources, including memory, life experience, self-expression, and knowledge, the occupational therapy practitioner can create an environment in which adaptive behaviors become learned skills. In return, the client takes an active part in the therapy process, contributing to the success of his or her own treatment. The responsibility of taking charge of one's health and well-being is reinforced through a cooperative process that allows the client to witness his or her own creative ability. Through this partnership, both the occupational therapy practitioner and the client validate the creative engagement that has occurred and gain an expectation that future creative adaptations can take place.

ACTIVITY 4-1

A limerick is a rhyming poem of five lines with the first, second, and fifth lines rhyming together and the third and fourth lines rhyming. For this task, write a limerick that describes the neuroscience of creativity or any part of the information in the module. The following are a few examples (Chudler, n.d.):

The brain uses neurons to think,
To know, to remember, to drink,
Without them you'll find,
You'll be in a bind,
Your body will fail and sink.

A neuron was once in the rain,
It said, "This is really a pain,"
It said to its friend,
"This must really end,"
So a message was sent to the brain.

The thalamus is a grand station,
It gives and receives information,
Gets messages here,
Sends messages there,
It's quite an important location.

The brain is important, that's true,
For all things a person will do,
From reading to writing,
To skiing to biting,
It makes up the person who's you.

It's a fortunate person whose brain
Is trained early, again and again,
And who continues to use it
To be sure not to lose it,
So the brain, in old age, may not wane.
(This last limerick was written by M. R. Rosenzweig and E. L. Bennett, in *Beh. Brain Res.,* 78:57-65, 1996)

ACTIVITY 4-2

Identify tasks, skills, or abilities in which you have participated and in which you believe you are well prepared. How have you used these tasks, skills, or abilities in creative ways?

ACTIVITY 4-3

Have a regular "creativity date." Set aside time each week or more or less often as you are able. The time allotted should be 2 to 4 hours. In that time, immerse yourself in an environment that nurtures creativity, visit a museum, art gallery, or nature center. Plan to watch a sunset or go to a concert. On the date, keep a journal or sketchbook and write or draw ideas that come to you. Write down stray thoughts or feelings without placing a value on them. Later, you can review the journal for inspiration for your creative endeavor, whether it is drawing, quilting, photography, writing, dance, or other creative activities.

QUESTIONS

1. What neurological evidence supports the idea that each of us can be creative?

2. How does this information about creativity affect your ability to develop long-term goals as a student? As an occupational therapy practitioner? As a client receiving occupational therapy?

3. When working with clients who have mental illness, how can this neurological information be used in planning treatment activities?

4. When working with elderly clients, what steps can be taken to help a person access long-term memory to solve problems in completing activities of daily living?

REFERENCES

Abraham, A., & Windmann, S. (2007). Creative cognition: The diverse operations and the prospect of applying a cognitive neuroscience perspective. *Methods, 42*(1), 38-48.

Baxter, D. A., & Byrne, J. H. (2006). Feeding behavior of *Aplysia*: A model system for comparing cellular mechanisms of classical and operant conditioning. *Learning & Memory, 13*(6): 669-680.

Bogousslavsky, J. (2005). Artistic creativity, style and brain disorders. *European Neurology, 54*(2), 103-111.

Buonomano, D. V., & Merzenich, M. M. (1998). Cortical plasticity: From synapses to maps. *Annual Review of Neuroscience, 21*, 149–186.

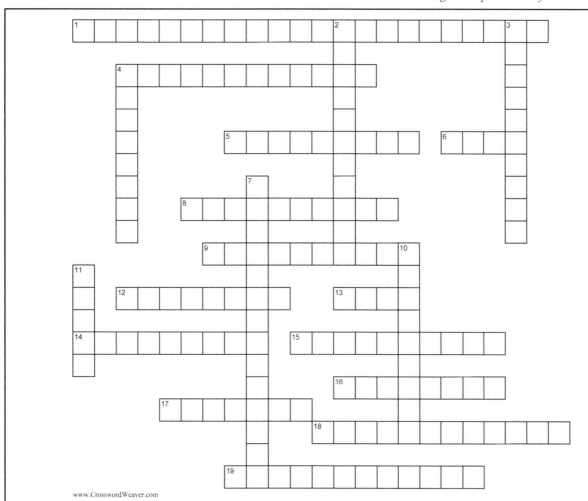

www.CrosswordWeaver.com

ACROSS

1 area of cortex that processes and integrates sensory information (2 words)

4 type of IQ which increases with experience and age

5 area of neocortex which stores domain specific knowledge

6 major inhibitory neurotransmitter of the brain

8 Released during creativity; processes calmness and a reduction in pain.

9 area of cortex responsible for working memory and attention

12 a creative person known for eccentricities related to tobacco.

13 a mental state experienced when fully immersed in an activity

14 _____ reserve; the mind's ability to resist damage to the brain

15 a period of time when ideas and directed thinking are set aside.

16 area of cortex; neural basis for higher cognitive functions

17 cognitive feature that is increased with creative activities and enriched contexts.

18 connects the limbic system with the autonomic nervous system

19 the confirmation of creative work by self or others

DOWN

2 the development of knowledge and skills

3 most abundant neurotransmitter in the CNS (2 words)

4 has been shown to inhibit focus; slows the thinking process and adds to depression

7 neurotransmitter reduced in creativity that allows memories to be ignored

10 a type of inhibition to incoming stimuli from the surrounding environment (2 words)

11 feature of the cortex which widens during aging, decreasing the brain surface

Cajal, R. S. (1916). *Advice for a young investigator*, (N. Swanson & L. Swanson, Trans.). Cambridge; The MIT Press.

Chakravarty, A. (2010). The creative brain - revisiting concepts. *Medical Hypotheses, 74*(3), 606-612.

Chatterjee, A. (2004). The neuropsychology of visual artistic production. *Neuropsychologia, 42*(11), 1568-1583.

Chermahini, S. A., & Hommel, B. (2010). The (b)link between creativity and dopamine: spontaneous eye blink rates predict and dissociate divergent and convergent thinking. *Cognition, 115*(2010), 458-465.

Chudler, E. H. (n.d.). Creative writing projects. Seattle, WA: Center for Sensorimotor Neural Engineering. Retrieved from http://faculty.washington.edu/chudler/writing.html

Csikszentmihalyi, M. (1997). *Finding Flow; The Psychology of Engagement with Everyday Life*. New York, NY: Basic Books.

Cummings, J. L., Miller, B. L., Christensen, D. D., & Cherry, D. (2008). Creativity and dementia: Emerging diagnostic and treatment methods for Alzheimer's disease. *CNS Spectrums, 13*(2 Suppl 2), 1-20; quiz 22.

Daykin, N., McClean, S., & Bunt, L. (2007). Creativity, identity and healing: Participants' accounts of music therapy in cancer care. *Health (London), 11*(3), 349-370.

Dietrich, A. (2004). The cognitive neuroscience of creativity. *Psychonomic Bulletin & Review, 11*(6), 1011-1026.

Dietrich, A. (2007). Who's afraid of a cognitive neuroscience of creativity? *Methods, 42*(1), 22-27.

Fink, A., Benedek, M., Grabner, R. H., Staudt, B., & Neubauer, A. C. (2007). Creativity meets neuroscience: Experimental tasks for the neuroscientific study of creative thinking. *Methods, 42*(1), 68-76.

Fink, A., Grabner, R. H., Benedek, M., Reishofer, G., Hauswirth, V., Fally, M., & Neubauer, A. C. (2009). The creative brain: Investigation of brain activity during creative problem solving by means of EEG and FMRI. *Human Brain Mapping, 30*(3), 734-748.

Heilman, K. M. (2005). *Creativity and the brain*. New York, NY: Psychology Press.

Heilman, K. M., Nadeau, S. E., & Beversdorf, D. O. (2003). Creative innovation: Possible brain mechanisms. *Neurocase: Case Studies in Neuropsychology, Neuropsychiatry, and Behavioural Neurology, 9*(5), 369-379.

Jung, R. E., Gasparovic, C., Chavez, R. S., Flores, R. A., Smith, S. M., Caprihan, A., & Yeo, R. A. (2009). Biochemical support for the "threshold" theory of creativity: A magnetic resonance spectroscopy study. *Journal of Neuroscience, 29*(16), 5319-5325.

Kalbfleisch, M. L. (2004). Functional neural anatomy of talent. *Anatomical Record. Part B, New Anatomist, 277*(1), 21-36.

Katz, A. N. (1979). Creativity and the cerebral hemispheres. *American Psychologist, 34*(3), 279-280.

Khasky, A. D., & Smith, J. C. (1999). Stress, relaxation states, and creativity. *Perceptual and Motor Skills, 88*(2), 409-416.

Kim, S., Hasher, L., & Zacks, R.T. (2008). Aging and a benefit of distractibility. Psychonomic Bulletin & Review, 14, 301-305.

Kowatari, Y., Lee, S. H., Yamamura, H., Nagamori, Y., Levy, P., Yamane, S., & Yamamoto, M. (2009). Neural networks involved in artistic creativity. *Human Brain Mapping, 30*(5), 1678-1690.

Kulisevsky, J., Pagonabarraga, J., & Martinez-Corral, M. (2009). Changes in artistic style and behaviour in Parkinson's disease: Dopamine and creativity. *Journal of Neurology, 256*(5), 816-819.

LeDoux, J. E. (2002). Synaptic self: How our brains become who we are. New York, NY: Viking.

Liu, A., Werner, K., Roy, S., Trojanowski, J. Q., Morgan-Kane, U., Miller, B. L., et al. (2009). A case study of an emerging visual artist with frontotemporal lobar degeneration and amyotrophic lateral sclerosis. *Neurocase, 15*(3), 235-247.

Mihov, K. M., Denzler, M., & Förster, J. (2010). Hemispheric specialization and creative thinking: A meta-analytic review of lateralization of creativity. *Brain and Cognition, 72*(3), 442-448.

Miller, B. L., Ponton, M., Benson, D. F., Cummings, J. L., & Mena, I. (1996). Enhanced artistic creativity with temporal lobe degeneration. *Lancet, 348*(9043), 1744-1745.

Mölle, M., Marshall, L., Lutzenberger, W., Pietrowsky, R., Fehm, H. L., & Born, J. (1996). Enhanced dynamic complexity in the human EEG during creative thinking. *Neuroscience Letters, 208*(1), 61-64.

Noice, H., Noice, T., & Staines, G. (2004) A short-term intervention to enhance cognitive and affective functioning in older adults. *Journal of Aging and Health, 16*(4):562-585.

Razoumnikova, O. M. (2000). Functional organization of different brain areas during convergent and divergent thinking: An EEG investigation. *Cognitive Brain Research, 10*(1-2), 11-18.

Sellal, F., & Musacchio, M. (2008). Artistic creativity and dementia. *Psychologie & Neuropsychiatrie Du Vieillissement, 6*(1), 57-66.

Taylor, I., & Taylor, M. M. (1990) *Psycholinguistics: Learning and using language*. Englewood Cliffs, NJ: Prentice-Hall.

Wallas, G. (1926). *The art of thought*. New York, NY: Harcourt Press.

Solution:

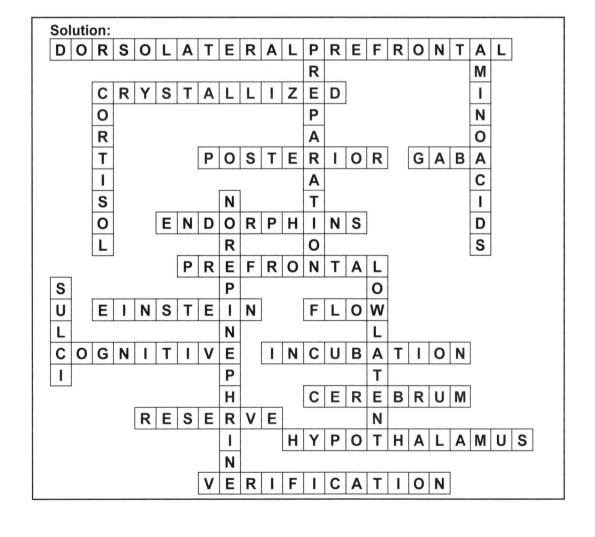

Benefits of Creativity: Building Professional Skills

Defining/identifying creativity

Recognizing/acknowledging use of creativity in OT

Describing the cognitive process of creativity

Understanding the neuroscience and structures of creativity

Incorporating creativity into professional skills

Applying creativity in client intervention

Applying research in creativity

5

Experiencing Creativity in the Learning Environment

Harriett A. Davidson, MA, OTR

The purpose of this chapter is to acknowledge the importance of learning environment in the development, characteristics, and outcomes of creativity. The learning environment and context include the academic setting and the field in which the student and practitioner work; for the client, they include the occupational therapy setting and the larger community and social system (Figure 5-1).

OBJECTIVES

1. Describe the features of a learning environment that fosters creativity.

2. Apply the principles of creative intervention involving activity analysis, grading, and adapting.

3. Explore methods of collaboration with clients for discovering creative solutions to clinical cases that present a challenge.

4. Describe the features of a creative learning environment.

5. Describe attributes of a creative learner's response to environmental challenges.

6. Explore four methods used in learning environments that foster creative responses.

7. Select personal learning environments and record their influence on your own creative responses.

8. Explain how the practice of grading and adapting fits into activity analysis, activity synthesis, and occupational analysis.

9. Explore innovative ways of conceptualizing the grading of activity and occupations as an individual's ability improves or diminishes.

10. Consider the client's readiness for collaborative creative problem solving.

11. Propose strategies for engaging clients in collaborative problem solving.

12. Identify cues that indicate a person's ability to collaborate in creative problem solving.

A culture of creativity is important. I am often inspired by works of art or ideas that are wildly different from my own. My brain wants to reinterpret things in a way that fits with my history. The more variety in those inspirations, the greater the leap into new thought. Feedback from others also strengthens or alters convictions about a creation. Often, a comment from someone sparks a new interpretation" (quote from a student asked to describe the ideal creative learning experience).

Coffey MS, Lamport NK, Hersch GI.
Creative Engagement in Occupation: Building Professional Skills (pp 61-71).
© 2015 SLACK Incorporated.

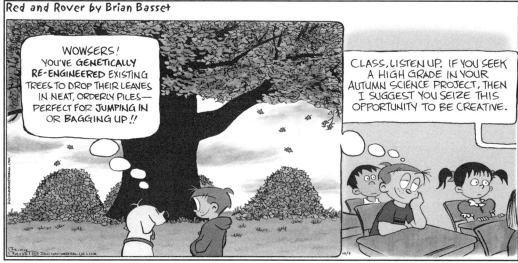

Unit 1: A Learning Environment That Fosters Creativity

The Culture of Creativity in Occupational Therapy Education and Practice

Since its inception, the field of occupational therapy has been described and experienced as one based on a person's ability to imagine and generate a rich array of alternative approaches to living life fully while simultaneously adapting to new situations. One question that a student entering an occupational therapy curriculum must answer is, "What will I be like as an occupational therapist?" Noted authors have described the artistic and scientific aspects of the field of occupational therapy (Abreu, 2011; Clark, 1993; Mosey, 1981a; Peloquin, 2005; Pierce, 2001), and the literature has depicted occupational therapists as skilled in both of them (Clark, 1993; Mosey, 1981b). Paterson, Higgs, and Donnelly (2012) described professional artistry as encompassing "the exceptional performance, actions, and behaviours of highly skilled, creative professional practitioners" (p. 95). Mosey (1981a) referred to the art of practice as "the capacity to establish rapport, to empathize, and to guide others to know and make use of their potential as participants in a community of others" (p. 4). Abreu, in her Slagle lecture, addressed the importance of empathy by saying, "In general, scholars have described empathy as a creative skill" (2011, p. 624). She elaborated on this principle as she fondly remembered a long career as an occupational therapist in which she "was able to use creativity

and imagination in therapy. The guiding question here was 'can we have fun today?'" (pp. 630-631).

The student's teacher in an occupational therapy curriculum can become a model for the use of creative interactions and relationships, commonly known in occupational therapy as *therapeutic use of self*. If the educational process teaches artistry and science, both of which demand creative approaches, then there can be an expectation to see evidence of both in the practice arena. Each curriculum for educating occupational therapy practitioners is organized according to selected values and theories about how people learn best. According to the *Occupational Therapy Model Curriculum* (OT Model Curriculum Ad Hoc Committee, 2008), a curriculum may be either *traditional* (or "rational") or *nontraditional* (or narrative). In both models, experiential learning is available to students following an Aristotelian model of "the things we have to learn before we can do them, we learn by doing them" (OTA Model Curriculum Committee, 2008). The educational environment that an occupational therapy student enters has been described in some of the professional literature and will be reviewed here.

Within the field of occupational therapy, at the individual course level, there is an instructor who brings a history of personal and educational experiences and acts as interpreter and integrator of the theory, knowledge, and skills that the student is expected to acquire. Hooper (2008) interviewed faculty members of an occupational therapy curriculum and analyzed their biographical experiences, their stated intentions for student formation, and the instructional processes they described. She found that they hoped to develop in their students a selective set of skills, including such things as "comfort with ambiguity," ability to "use observations to generate new evidence," and "...find a connection [with a research topic] and figure out how they can insert themselves into the spaces that are wide open" (pp. 232-234). In other words, these faculty members seem to be saying that they want to help students develop elements of creativity.

How faculty members define and give meaning to the term *creativity* may vary. Kleiman (2008) reported the results of a phenomenographic study of university lecturers from the arts, humanities, and sciences in England, in which they were asked to describe the meaning of creativity in learning and teaching. The results revealed different meanings of creativity, variously focused on constraint, process, product, transformation, and fulfillment. Therefore, the learner may find that the expectations of each instructor are different and that the learning atmosphere he or she encounters is different for each curriculum.

The challenge to students in an occupational therapy curriculum is to learn the sound principles of occupational science while using their imagination and the time to achieve implementation of those principles. Students will evaluate their instructors' actions and attempt to understand, engage, and incorporate the knowledge and skills (including those related to creativity) offered by them. In some ways, this process parallels how the client receiving occupational therapy will consider the practitioner's intentions and actions and accept or reject them, interpret or misinterpret them. The occupational therapy classroom reflects the culture of occupational therapy, as personified by the faculty members, the learning activities, and the students. The occupational therapy clinic reflects this culture as well, as personified by the practitioners, the treatment activities, and the clients.

Features of the Creative Learning Environment

Of course, the education for and practice of occupational therapy rely on what might be called *creative knowledge environments* (Hemlin, Allwood, & Martin, 2008). The following features have been identified as important in a rich creative learning environment and, when found within an occupational therapy learning setting, can provide an opportunity for experiencing creativity. They also can provide models that students can put into practice.

Culturally Diverse Ideas

Multicultural experience has been shown to result in creative outcomes and processes, "especially when people adapt and are open to these new experiences and when the creative context deemphasizes the need for firm answers" (Leung, Maddux, Galinsky, & Chiu,

2008, p. 177). Multicultural experience need not involve traveling to another country, although that can be an important influence on creativity. In a typical occupational therapy curriculum, students from a variety of backgrounds, representing many different cultures and ideas, are enrolled; thus, each student brings his or her own unique culture.

In addition to outside cultural experiences, the culture of occupational therapy can benefit from interacting with those of other disciplines within the educational or practice setting (e.g., physical therapy, psychology, nursing, nutrition and food science, health care administration, architecture, mathematics, physics, and biology). When solving a problem, developing a treatment, or understanding task analysis, for instance, the benefits of interacting with students of mathematics or physics can include enhanced discovery and innovation. Three methods of learning that are commonly found in occupational therapy curricula also share the opportunity to experience cultural diversity: service learning, learning through discussion (LTD), and team-based learning. These methods are described more fully later in this chapter.

Opportunities for a Variety of Therapeutic Styles

Taylor (2008), in her work on the intentional relationship, attempted to describe the style of occupational therapists who were identified as personifying the ideal therapeutic relationship and found many different adjectives given by many people, such as energetic, positive, playful, spontaneous, reliable, caring, and giving. She concluded that different styles are important for different situations and for different practice areas, with the creative use of self and situation being the foremost consideration.

Respect for Students' Integrity and Freedom to Explore Learner-Centered Approaches

In general, occupational therapy students are accustomed to "learning through doing" and are active learners. This approach asks students to take responsibility for their own learning and to share it equally with the teacher. Teachers are careful to "focus on all aspects of learning and the learning process, as opposed to teaching" (Kramer et al., 2007, p. 186).

Atmosphere of a Creative Learning Environment

A creative learning environment might elicit some of the following characteristics in learners (derived from Csikszentmihalyi's [1996] studies of flow):

Curiosity in a place where things are happening and there are opportunities to continue learning

Spontaneity in a climate of innovation with the opportunity to look everywhere for inspiration

Pleasure from a multicultural/interdisciplinary environment in which diversity is welcome and celebrated

Humor found with tolerance for different teaching-learning styles and opportunities for risk taking and failure

Creativity expanded when faced with a hive of ideas, new languages, and approaches with values that force reconsideration and expansion of thinking and practice

One example of a dynamic curriculum design is requiring an elective course in a subject outside of one's field (e.g., a cooking class) to evaluate discoveries through projects, equally important as exams, and to self-correct when given feedback from peers or the instructor.

Attributes of Creative Learners' Responses to Environmental Challenges

In examining the attributes that follow, a creative learner can be the occupational therapy student, the practitioner, or the client who is likely to willingly respond to the following demands.

Problem Solving

The student has the stamina to systematically wrestle with a problem until a solution is reached (and then test that solution for a successful outcome). In a similar way, the client receiving occupational therapy is able to try different ways of accomplishing a task despite fatigue (until finding one that works).

Clinical Reasoning

The student is intrigued by the puzzles presented in classroom activities and by clinical situations and recognizes with confidence the capacity to work through the questions. The client can understand that continuing an enabling activity (e.g., involving use of the hands) will help him or her regain the skill to complete some aspect of a chosen occupation, such as diapering a baby.

Critical Thinking

The student is encouraged and willing to tackle hard questions and willing to consider alternative interpretations and then defend his or her own position while balancing the ability to imagine creative possibilities. The occupational therapy practitioner may discern that the temporary use of adaptive equipment for this client may help him or her gain some independence sooner and can be set aside when strength returns.

Risk Taking

When the creative learner is working in an atmosphere that is trusting, safe, and supportive, he or she is enabled to take the risks that are inherent in the creative process. Recall that the creativity process has been described as having four stages: preparation, incubation, illumination, and verification. Although the student has the opportunity to learn new and stimulating information, within the creative process there is uncertainty of the outcome, i.e., there is a risk that actions or events may not turn out the way expected or desired. This potential can produce both anxiety and excitement. For example, if students or clients are led to feel that they must succeed in a venture the first time they try it, then creativity can be inhibited.

Understanding Basic Principles

Creative innovations come about when one first understands and has mastered the basic principles of the subject under study. For example, a practitioner with a background in physical principles of the hand, including the potential movement planes and patterns, can study objects with comparable properties and then design a splint that assists hand position, movement, or sensation for a specific client.

Methods Used in Educational Environments That Foster Creative Responses

Certain learning methods that occupational therapy curricula typically use are designed to elicit creative responses. Kramer et al. (2007) described a learner-centered curriculum model designed to develop "engagement, critical thinking, innovations in practice, and clinical reasoning" in occupational therapy students (p. 185). Four methods were incorporated in the curriculum and studied: service learning, LTD, team-based learning, and sequential design of research coursework.

Service Learning

Service learning is a method that involves students interfacing with agencies in a variety of community settings to work in partnership with a diverse group of individuals and cultures. It provides an opportunity to develop interpersonal skills, foster critical thinking about real community issues, and explore innovations in practice. A trend toward increased creative thinking and problem solving by students was found to occur in this type of learning environment.

Learning Through Discussion

LTD is a method of learning that relies on a structured plan, group dynamics, and an in-depth study of the material. Originally designed to encourage critical analysis, it allows for the systematic sharing of viewpoints of all members of the discussion group, which can set the stage for the possible emergence of new and creative insights into the material being discussed. The process, originally developed by Hill (1962) and updated by Rabow, Charness, Kipperman, and Radcliffe-Vasile (1994), involves the following eight steps: (1) checking in; (2) learning the vocabulary; (3) hearing a general statement of the author's message; (4) identifying and discussing the major themes or subtopics; (5) applying the material to other works; (6) applying the material to self; (7) evaluating the author's presentation; and (8) evaluating group and individual performance (Rabow et al., p. 40). By step eight, one might assume that the group arrives at a common conclusion. However, it is the fourth step that produces a rich flow of ideas, filtered through the mind of each group member, and prompts new ways of thinking by the participants. The culture represented by each person in the group enriches the interpretation and outcome of the discussion.

In the LTD environment, students take responsibility for studying the material and for leading reflective discussions, which provides an opportunity to consider many viewpoints and potential solutions to the issues at hand. Each member of the group starts with an article or text that reports research or a document of some merit. A dynamic context is provided for sharing ideas, venturing to explore them, daring to propose new interpretations, and creating an environment with ideas flowing freely. No judgments are made about the "goodness" of the ideas; all of them are worthy of consideration. Rabow, Charness, Kipperman, and Radcliffe-Vasile (1994) reported increased critical thinking and clinical reasoning with the use of this type of learning environment.

Team-Based Learning

This method involves more than just group learning; it is a sharing of goals and diversity of roles, and it directs attention to the dynamics of the group. The team has an assigned task related to the classroom content. Kramer et al. (2007) reported increased critical thinking and clinical reasoning with use of this method. For examples of team-based learning, see the work by Collins, Harrison, Mason, and Lowden (2011) and Murray (2010).

Structured Research Course

These courses provide a disciplined look at the background of a study topic and encourage knowing that topic well through rigorous research protocol. New discoveries are possible, and the design and grading criteria can allow for creativity (Kramer et al., 2007).

ACTIVITY 5-1

To examine your own personal learning environment and the influence of your creative responses, create a "creative events" timeline for the previous month. Begin by delineating when and where your classes or work periods occurred. Then, include when and where study or reflection times happened. Look at your own course syllabus or completed work to note when and where you experienced significant creativity. Retrospectively identify on your timeline when you had an "aha" moment. Was it when the original idea was developed or when you recognized it as a good or not-good idea? Compare your timeline with that of a peer to discover whether the same class or experience elicited the same or a different creative response. Note the variety of creative responses reported.

ACTIVITY 5-2

To compare the creative outcome accomplished in a solitary setting with one completed in a group with four other students, all working on the same project, create a game that will teach senior citizens in a long-term care facility about what occupational therapy can do to benefit them.

First, create the game by yourself. Then, create another game with a group of four other students. Develop a set of criteria for comparing your results, and examine how the games were similar and different from each other.

ACTIVITY 5-3

You should now be ready to design your own experiment. Given a learning task of your own invention, choose one of two learning environments (solitary or group oriented) to use for producing creativity in the outcomes. Noting when each stage of the creative process occurs is important (review Chapter 3 to recall the four stages: preparation, incubation, illumination, and verification).

If the learning task involves "hatching" an idea, you might want to look at the natural world around you to see how nature has solved some problems. For example, "the sticky hook spine of the common burr inspired the man who invented Velcro fastener" (von Oech, 1990, p. 110).

You might go for a walk in the woods or along the seashore. Are there suggestions you might find for designing a game for a client with sensory-motor difficulties? For a client who needs an assistive device to store and transport items? For a client with cognitive difficulties to develop strategies for memory assistance or for rest and sleep?

- What kinds of shapes can you find by watching the ocean waves? What kinds of actions?

- How many different kinds of footprints/imprints do you find in the sand, and what made each of them?

- How do the vines growing up the trees hang on or attach themselves? What differences do you see in the patterns of leaves from two or more kinds of trees?

- Do any of these things suggest patterns to help you in designing the answer to your problem?

If you selected a method for implementing an idea you have, you might want to look for a setting in which you might see the use of a similar principle or strategy applied to a different activity or product. One can benefit from studying and interacting not only with other disciplines in the academic or the health care setting but also within the community at large. For example, what can you learn about movement and perception from taking a modern dance class? To implement an idea for another problem you are trying to solve, you might do the following:

- Go to an auto repair shop
- Go to a children's playground
- Go to an animal shelter

What processes, people, or activities are suggested by what you see that might be applied to the implementation of your idea?

UNIT 2: PRINCIPLES OF CREATIVE INTERVENTIONS INVOLVING ACTIVITY ANALYSIS, GRADING, AND ADAPTING

Through the activity analysis process, the student gains some experience with *grading* and *adapting*. These processes are critically important aspects of occupational therapy practice. Crepeau and Schell (2009) remind us that *activity analysis* is the way that occupational therapists think about activities. It is a tool for designing interventions so that demands can be increased to improve performance or, conversely, demands can be decreased to match a person's diminishing ability to perform a task. Activity analysis is also a therapist's way of selecting potential activities to promote therapeutic goals for clients. This analysis provides a powerful tool for designing a best fit between what the individual wants to do and needs to do and can do. Therefore, grading and adapting are the tools for designing the *activity synthesis*, or the match between a client's current abilities and his or her desired participation in an activity or occupation, and for planning future changes in the individual's performance. Indeed, each person does this every day. Crepeau and Schell refer to this synthesis of information from the client's occupational profile to address selected occupations within context as *occupational analysis* (2009, p. 369). "Grading means to arrange or position in a scale of size, quality, or intensity. Grading can be compared to measuring how much of a specific task is performed" (Hersch, Lamport, & Coffey, 2005, p. 63). Hersch et al. point out that every activity that an occupational therapy practitioner uses in intervention should be gradable so that the client's progress can be documented.

One method of grading can be performed in terms of the level of skill and the seriousness of the meaning of the activity to the individual. In *Model of Human Occupation*, Kielhofner (2002) articulated how a client can go through the following three progressive stages of occupation: exploration, competency, and achievement. During the *exploration stage*, activities can be playful, and there is no penalty for failure; this stage can allow a client to experiment with the materials, objects, or ideas being manipulated and managed and the space and contextual features acting upon the situation. This, in turn, may allow for the incubation phase of creativity. During the *competency stage*, the individual is wrestling fully with the elements of the task, object, or procedure. Until competency is reached, the next step—achievement—may not occur. Kielhofner calls this final stage the *achievement stage*. When competency is reached, it may lead to the intended outcome or into directions not anticipated. As an example, the clear goal of Edward Jenner was to cure smallpox. When he came to the understanding that he did not have the tools to accomplish that goal, he turned from his original focus to look at people who did not contract smallpox. He discovered that these people had had cowpox, and this research led to his ability to produce a vaccine to prevent smallpox (von Oech, 1990, p. 144).

Another term that is important in occupational therapy when assisting clients toward full participation in an occupation is *adaptation*. One definition of adaptation found in the *OTPF* (Second Edition) is "the response approach the client makes encountering an occupational challenge" (American Occupational Therapy Association, 2008, p. 669). Schultz and Schkade further explain that "this change is implemented when the individual's customary response approaches are found inadequate for producing some degree of mastery over the challenge" (1997, p. 474). Therapeutic adaptations may involve designing or restructuring the client's physical environment to assist with performing occupations successfully. This may also include instructing the client, family, or caregiver in the proper use, maintenance, modification, or minor repair of the equipment involved. The goal of adaptation is to make it possible for the person to engage in a valued occupation rather than to change the skill level of the person (Crepeau & Schell, 2009, pp. 368-371). An outcome of therapeutic intervention may be the modification of a behavior or redesign of a strategy for accomplishing an occupational task, or it may be the availability of an assistive device or method (American Occupational Therapy Association, p. 662). A person may be able to experience relative mastery of a task, as indicated by that person's qualitative appraisal of efficiency, effectiveness, and satisfaction for him- or herself and for others (Schultz, 2014, p. 532).

ACTIVITY 5-4

To explore potential adaptations when a performance skill is no longer intact, tape the thumb of your dominant hand down into a position in which it cannot be used. Then, try to perform activities using just your other four fingers (e.g., send a text message, make pancakes, or apply your make-up). What adaptations did you make because you were working with four digits and no opposing thumb?

Now, do the same activity with your nondominant hand. What different adaptations were effective?

ACTIVITY 5-5

To explore innovative ways of conceptualizing grading activities and occupations as an individual's ability improves or diminishes, identify models and metaphors from other disciplines. For example:

- From physics: an inclined plane
- From architecture: stair steps, with each step equal to the next one in size and height
- From the world of play: a merry-go-round accelerating over time

- From agriculture: more leaves appearing on a branch over time
- From horticulture: a rose with petals opening gradually
- From exercise physiology: more metabolic equivalents, more reps, more time, more distance

ACTIVITY 5-6

Using Worksheet 5-1, select an activity and apply creative thinking to the task of grading and adapting in different ways, as directed in the instructions.

UNIT 3: EXPLORING METHODS OF CLIENT COLLABORATION TO DISCOVER CREATIVE SOLUTIONS

Consider Readiness of the Client for Collaborative Creative Problem Solving

A client may resist trying to do new things because the need for change is not evident or because of a belief that his or her disabling condition is reversible. Conversely, there may be a loss of hope and no psychic energy available for creativity. The client may have a belief system that dictates that a condition should be accepted without protest. There may be a cultural assumption that it is another person's responsibility to assume the roles the client relinquished to take on the role of a person with a disability. Or, there may be a physical, cognitive, or sensory loss that does not permit the client to continue with his or her usual creative engagement. Crepeau and Schell (2009) remind us that the occupational therapy practitioner's role in grading may be to alter the task by gradually increasing or decreasing demands, but other roles in the process may appear—to scaffold (assist with the too-hard parts), to fade (withdraw assistance as the client's ability grows), or to coach (provide verbal and emotional support as needed) (p. 367).

Propose Strategies for Engaging the Client in Collaborative Problem Solving

Occupational therapy practitioners may use a variety of the interpersonal strategies identified in Taylor's (2008) research on the therapeutic process. She speaks of developing an intentional relationship with clients and advocates six specific therapeutic modes (p. 68). How one uses these strategies depends on the style that is comfortable to the individual and also relies on a skillful understanding of the occasion and the needs of the client at that moment. Taylor labeled these modes *advocating, collaborating, empathizing, encouraging, instructing,* and *problem solving.* The art of matching the style to the client's need and the situation must involve sensitivity and creativity. In the advocating mode (pp. 69-72), the therapist works on behalf of the client to determine whether the needed resources are available for the client to participate in all areas of life. In the collaborating mode (pp. 74-75), the therapist takes an egalitarian approach, expecting the client to participate actively in therapy. In the empathizing mode (pp. 75-78), the therapist listens carefully and attempts to fully understand the client's communication. In the encouraging mode (pp. 78-81), the therapist works to instill courage, hope, and the will to explore further. In the instructing mode (pp. 80-81), the therapist becomes a teacher, being logical and instructive. And, in the problem-solving mode (pp. 81-82), the therapist approaches the situation with the client reasonably and logically.

Benefits of Creativity in Occupational Therapy Education and in Practice

Occupational therapy students encounter new principles, theories, models, guidelines, and precautions through their coursework. Once these principles are learned, the student must incorporate them into practice. Being involved as a student in the exploration and understanding of the creative process can help one's growth as an occupational therapist.

In 1965, Torrance defined creativity as "the process of becoming sensitive to problems, deficiencies, gaps in knowledge, missing elements, disharmonies, and so on…" (p. 663). He elaborated the process by describing the search for solutions and the development and testing of hypotheses. Later literature, of course, added the notions of utility and value to the definition of creativity (Kleiman, 2008). The process just described can lead to new tools and new outcomes that occupational therapy as a profession can use to survive and prosper. On the basis of the work of Blanche (2008), Kuhaneck, Spitzer, and Miller (2010) made the argument that developing creativity can help one to "better meet the challenges of practice" (p. 64).

Taylor (2008) stated that when building an interpersonal skill base, the therapist (unless using a highly structured interview protocol) should become skilled at asking questions creatively. She recommended "Changing the sequence of questions, rephrasing them, or asking them in more creative ways that match the client's interpersonal needs of the moment" (p. 198). Involving the client in the creative process represents a client-centered approach, to the extent the client is able to participate. The practitioner and the client creating an evaluation and intervention plan jointly is, in itself, a creative process. Besides the client learning self-awareness and self-management, there is evidence that there can be improved follow-through of the intervention and outcomes (Carswell et al., 2004). Some literature has suggested that playfulness, which contains an important creativity component, supports wellness and resiliency (Metzl & Morrell, 2008). This idea deserves more testing and study, and there is growing evidence to support the healthful benefits of playfulness and creativity (Guitard, Ferland, & Dutil, 2005).

By being provided all the features of a creative environment and applying the personal attributes of a creative learner, clients can participate in creative problem solving during their treatment. Students can continue to learn from classroom experiences and outside influences while developing into creative occupational therapy practitioners. Faculty members will model and teach, and students can gain insight by observing the ways in which they are taught; they can adopt, adapt, try out, or reject their instructors' ideas and tactics as they see fit, according to their own styles.

ACTIVITY 5-7

Given the following case, in which the client is nonverbal and the potential for creative responses is unknown, suggest methods for determining the client's ability to respond in any manner (refer to information from the previous chapters on cognition and neuroscience to recall some ways in which Mrs. Rose might be able to respond):

Mrs. Rose is an 88-year-old woman who comes into your clinic in a wheelchair, and you discover that she has severe aphasia as a result of a stroke. She makes good eye contact and sits while waiting for you to speak. Which of Taylor's modes might you use for your initial approach, and what possible responses might you elicit from Mrs. Rose? How would you set up a learning environment for Mrs. Rose to create an atmosphere conducive for her to participate in her therapy?

Conclusion

In this chapter, some of the approaches and ideas for creating a learning environment to foster the use of creativity have been identified. Understanding learners' needs and strategies for encouraging creativity in performing everyday tasks has been highlighted. The aspects of risk taking, therapeutic use of self, grading, and adaptation have been explored in the context of engaging clients in their occupational therapy. Continuing this process of observing, recognizing, and attempting to use creativity in treatment planning is building an important professional skill.

Questions

1. What is the most creative thing you did this year? Where did you do it? What did you learn from it?

2. What are some ways in which a therapist can tap creativity in a client spontaneously (or with modeling and teaching)?

3. Are there readiness points in yourself for developing creative approaches to learning new occupational skills and routines? How can you apply this knowledge to your clients' situations?

4. If you look at the history of creative advances, you will find examples of failed efforts at discovery (recall the story of Edward Jenner in his attempt to cure smallpox). Have you had experience with creativity that did not turn out as you had hoped? How did you deal with it?

5. Consider a client whose expectation is to return home at discharge, but the reality is that his health status requires caregiving in an assisted living facility rather than an independent setting. How would you make it possible for your client to "therapeutically fail" and come to this conclusion creatively?

References

Abreu, B. C. (2011). Accentuate the positive: Reflections on empathic interpersonal interactions. *American Journal of Occupational Therapy, 65*(6), 623-634.

American Occupational Therapy Association. (2008). Occupational therapy practice framework: Domain & process (2nd ed.) *American Journal of Occupational Therapy, 62*(6), 625-683.

Blanche, E. I. (2008). Play in children with cerebral palsy: Doing with—not doing to. In L. D. Parham, & L. S. Fazio (Eds.), *Play in occupational therapy for children* (2nd ed., pp. 375-393). St. Louis, MO: Mosby Elsevier.

Carswell, A., McColl, M., Baptiste, S., Law, M., Polatajko, H., & Pollock, N. (2004). The Canadian Occupational Performance Measure: A research and clinical literature review. *Canadian Journal of Occupational Therapy, 71*(4), 210-222.

Clark, F. (1993). Occupation embedded in real life: Interweaving occupational science and occupational therapy. *American Journal of Occupational Therapy, 47*(12), 1067-1077.

Collins, M., Harrison, D., Mason, R., & Lowden, S. (2011). Innovation and creativity: Exploring human occupation and professional development in student education. *British Journal of Occupational Therapy, 74*(6), 304-308.

Crepeau, E. B., & Schell, B. A. B. (2009). Analyzing occupations and activity. In E. B. Crepeau, E. S. Cohn, & B. A. B. Schell (Eds.). *Willard & Spackman's occupational therapy* (11th ed.). Baltimore, MD: Lippincott Williams & Wilkins.

Csikszentmihalyi, M. (1996). *Flow and the psychology of innovation.* New York, NY: HarperCollins.

Guitard, P., Ferland, F., & Dutil, E. (2005). Toward a better understanding of playfulness in adults. *OTJR: Occupation, Participation and Health, 25*(1), 9-22.

Hemlin, S., Allwood, C. M., & Martin, B. R. (2008). Creative knowledge environments. *Creativity Research Journal, 20*(2), 196-210.

Hersch, G. I., Lamport, N. K., & Coffey, M. S. (2005). *Activity analysis: Application to occupation* (5th ed.). Thorofare, NJ: SLACK Incorporated.

Hill, W. F. (1962). *Learning through discussion.* Long Grove, IL: Waveland Press.

Hooper, B. (2008). Stories we teach by: Intersections among faculty biography, student formation and instructional processes. *American Journal of Occupational Therapy, 62*(2), 228-241.

Kielhofner, G. (2002). *Model of human occupation* (3rd ed.). Baltimore, MD: Lippincott Williams & Wilkins.

Kleiman, P. (2008). Towards transformation: Conceptions of creativity in higher education. *Innovations in Education and Teaching International, 45*(3), 209-217.

Kramer, P., Ideishi, R., Kearney, P., Cohen, M., Ames, J., Shea, G., Schemm, R., & Blumberg, P. (2007). Achieving curricular themes through learning-centered teaching. *Occupational Therapy in Health Care, 21*(1/2), 185-198.

Kuhaneck, H. M., Spitzer, S. L., & Miller, E. (2010). *Activity analysis, creativity, and playfulness in pediatric occupational therapy.* Boston, MA: Jones and Bartlett.

Leung, A. K., Maddux, W. W., Galinsky, A. D., & Chiu, C. (2008). Multicultural experience enhances creativity. *American Psychologist, 63*(3), 169-181.

Metzl, E. S., & Morrell, M. A. (2008). The role of creativity in models of resilience: Theoretical exploration and practical applications. *Journal of Creativity in Mental Health, 3*(3), 303-318.

Mosey, A. C. (1981a). Introduction: The art of practice. In B. C. Abreu (Ed.), *Physical disabilities manual* (pp. 1-3). New York, NY: Raven.

Mosey, A. C. (1981b). *Occupational therapy: Configuration of a profession.* New York, NY: Raven Press.

Murray, C. (2010). Fostering student creativity. *OT Practice Magazine, 15*(17), 9-12.

Paterson, M., Higgs, J., & Donnelly, C. (2012). Artistry and expertise. In L. Robertson (Ed.), *Clinical reasoning in occupational therapy: Controversies in practice.* Chichester, West Sussex, UK: Wiley-Blackwell.

Pierce, D. (2001). Occupation by design: Dimensions, therapeutic power, and creative process. *American Journal of Occupational Therapy, 55*(3), 249-259.

Peloquin, S. M. (2005). Embracing our ethos, reclaiming our heart. *American Journal of Occupational Therapy, 59*(6), 611-625.

OT Model Curriculum Ad Hoc Committee. (2008). *Occupational therapy model curriculum.* Rockville, MD: American Occupational Therapy Association.

OTA Model Curriculum Committee (2008). *Occupational therapy assistant model curriculum.* Rockville, MD: American Occupational Therapy Association.

Rabow, J., Charness, M. A., Kipperman, J., & Radcliffe-Vasile, S. (1994). *William Fawcett Hill's learning through discussion* (3rd ed.). Thousand Oaks, CA: Sage.

Schultz, S., & Schkade, J. (1997). Adaptation. In C. Christiansen, & M. C. Baum (Eds.), *Occupational therapy: Enabling function and well-being* (p. 474). Thorofare, NJ: SLACK Incorporated.

Schultz, S. W. (2014). Theory of occupational adaptation. In B. A. B. Schell, G. Gillen, & M. E. Scaffa (Eds.), In *Willard & Spackman's occupational therapy* (12th ed., pp. 527-540). Baltimore, MD: Lippincott Williams & Wilkins.

Taylor, R. R. (2008). *The intentional relationship: Occupational therapy and use of self.* Philadelphia, PA: F. A. Davis.

Torrance, E. P. (1965). Scientific views of creativity and factors affecting its growth. *Daedalus, 95*(3), 663-681.

von Oech, R. (1990). *A whack on the side of the head* (Rev. ed.). Stamford, CT: U.S. Games Systems.

Worksheet 5-1

Grading and Adapting an Activity

Student: _____   Activity: _____   Date: _____

Describe an activity in several sentences to give an overview of how you perform it normally (for example, "I tie a bow on a present using both hands in different ways. My dominant hand [right] is used to hold the strand of ribbon and wrap it around the box while my nondominant hand holds the position of the box. I place my left index finger over the knot, applying pressure to hold it as I loop the ribbon into a bow and tie it using my right hand.")

State one way to grade this activity in terms of the performance skills required to make it more simple or more complex (indicate which):

1. Someone with a limited attention span:

2. Someone with limited endurance and/or strength in both arms:

State one way to adapt this activity so that those who are unable to perform it in the usual way can succeed by performing the same activity with the same outcome.

1. Someone with limited use of one or both hands:

2. Someone with limited vision:

Benefits of Creativity: Building Professional Skills
Defining/identifying creativity
Recognizing/acknowledging use of creativity in OT
Describing the cognitive process of creativity
Understanding the neuroscience and structures of creativity
Incorporating creativity into professional skills
Applying creativity in client intervention
Applying research in creativity

6

Experiencing Creativity in Client Intervention

Gayle I. Hersch, PhD, OTR

"It sounded an excellent plan, no doubt, and very neatly and simply arranged; the only difficulty was, she had not the smallest idea how to set about it."

Lewis Carroll, *Alice's Adventures in Wonderland* (1865, p. 37)

This chapter asks students to experience the process of discovering their own creative potential and of problem solving to develop creative interventions for clients.

OBJECTIVES

1. Trace the use of creativity in the profession of occupational therapy.

2. Describe the connection of client-centered practice with creativity.

3. Tap into your own creative potential.

4. Appreciate the use of occupational analysis in thinking creatively.

5. Use various ways of thinking creatively.

6. Apply the occupational performance analysis process to think creatively.

7. Describe the language of occupational therapy as characterized by the most recent *Occupational Therapy Practice Framework* (*OTPF*) (American Occupational Therapy Association [AOTA], 2008) and its components.

8. Apply the language of occupational therapy (e.g., areas of occupation, body functions, performance skills/patterns) in analyzing activities creatively.

9. Problem solve creatively to achieve occupation-based client interventions.

10. Develop creative therapeutic interventions for a variety of adults of different ages.

11. Value creativity and its application in the therapeutic process.

Coffey MS, Lamport NK, Hersch GI.
Creative Engagement in Occupation: Building Professional Skills (pp 73-96).

Important Terms

Client-centered practice
Creative potential
Occupational performance
Occupational analysis
Creative client intervention

Unit 1: Rationale for Infusing Creativity Into Practice

This unit offers justification for and explanation of the experiential activities in which the student will engage.

Infusing Creativity Into Current and Future Practice

Where is creativity in occupational therapy? How does it come about? What can I do to make it happen? Students reading this text will begin by asking these questions, especially after studying the previous chapters about the definition of creativity, its foundation in occupational therapy, its neurological base and cognitive implications, and its therapeutic value and application in practice. This chapter attempts to help each student respond to these questions and begin to feel comfortable tapping into his or her own creativity.

Perrin (2001) challenges us to return to the art of using occupations as therapy and appreciating the lost art of infusing creativity into our daily client practice. She offers the "fluffy bunny syndrome" to demonstrate how our therapeutic tools are commonplace. Yet, when applied creatively and for a specific client goal, they can be the reason for a successful outcome. She asserts that the creativity of the therapeutic relationship has been lost to standard reimbursement-ensured protocols in which clients have no choice or control over what is included in the treatment regime. In contrast, in a client-centered practice, the client is an active participant in the formulation of a new solution/treatment regime. "A creative drive towards a new 'product' must be at the heart of every therapeutic intervention" (Perrin, p. 132).

According to Fromm (1959), four conditions are essential for tapping into one's own creativity. First, have an attitude of wonder, curiosity, and questioning; second, accept, even welcome and appreciate, the conflicts that arise in life; third, be single-minded and absorbed in the here and now; and fourth, embrace the unknown future by letting go of the past. In other words, creativity is spurred by engaging in the environment and making something that we can claim as our own.

In Schmid's (2005) text on promoting health through creativity, she defined creativity as "the innate capacity to think and act in original ways, to be inventive, to be imaginative and to find new and original solutions to needs, problems, and forms of expression. It can be used in all activities. Its processes and outcomes are meaningful to its user and generate positive feelings" (p. 29). By experiencing the creative process, the student will discover that the result or the end product is meaningful and elicits satisfaction.

Tapping Into Your Creative Potential

Worksheets 6-1 through 6-3 are intended to have you think about the ways in which creativity has been described and applied by occupational therapists and reflect on your own creative potential. Worksheet 6-1 asks for you to critique two articles from the occupational therapy literature; Worksheet 6-2 allows you to become aware of your creativity from a past situation; and Worksheet 6-3 asks you to journal your creativity as you progress through the academic program/course.

Unit 2: Analyzing Occupational Performance Creatively

The purpose of this unit is to have the student apply the process of occupational analysis to thinking creatively. Worksheets will guide students through the process of analyzing occupational performance creatively as they perform activities.

Thinking Creatively

When asked the question, "Are you creative?" most people will say "not really" or "sometimes I have a moment of genius." How would you respond? Can you think of a time when you felt and thought that you were being creative or thinking creatively? How would you describe it?

One of the first models to describe the creative process was offered by Graham Wallas (1926). In the Wallas model, creative insights and illuminations were explained by a process consisting of the following five stages:

1. *Preparation* (preparatory work is done on a problem that focuses the individual's mind on the problem and explores the problem's dimensions)

2. *Incubation* (the problem is internalized in the unconscious mind and nothing appears to be happening externally)

3. *Intimation* (the creative person gets a feeling that a solution is on its way)

4. *Illumination* or insight (the creative idea bursts forth from its preconscious processing into conscious awareness)

5. *Verification* (the idea is consciously verified, elaborated, and applied)

A second technique for tapping into creativity is called *mapping* (Michalko, 2006; provided by Michael Michalko with permission for use in this text [2/13/2012 electronic communication]). Mapping a challenge is designed to help you communicate with yourself. First, think of a challenge you currently have. Then, jot down whatever thoughts you have about that challenge. It is ok if these thoughts are loose, disconnected, and incomplete. Organize them on paper by placing them wherever you think they belong or where they don't fit. Study the map. If no ideas come after prolonged study, you will probably feel uneasy. In that case, put the map away for a few days. When you return to it, you should find that your mind is more focused on the challenge, and you will usually experience a moment of insight. This should be followed by a period of concentrated thought, during which the insight unfolds into a complete idea.

To further map your ideas, use the graphic technique of *think bubbles* for organizing your thoughts. Create an actual, physical picture of how your mind dissects a challenge and manipulates the bits of information to arrive at a solution.

Although maps can and should be highly individualized, all mind maps share the following four basic characteristics (Provided by Michael Michalko with permission for use in this text [2/13/2012 electronic communication]):

1. *Organization.* Mapping presents information organized in the way you think of it. It displays the way your mind works, complete with patterns and interrelationships, and it has an amazing capacity to convey precise information, no matter how crudely drawn. You can make your map of think bubbles as simple or as complex as you want. You can use a large sheet of paper, a blackboard, or anything you like. You can group related ideas of equal importance horizontally and use connecting arrows to denote special relationships or color code different types of relationships. The visual, flexible nature of mapping makes it extremely useful as a device to help us see, express, and think about complex problems. You can readily add to the map later, and you should be prepared to do so, because your first map will rarely produce an idea that meets all of your criteria.

2. *Key words.* Ignore all irrelevant words and phrases and concentrate only on expressing the essentials and what associations they excite in your mind.

3. *Association.* Make connections, links, and relationships between seemingly isolated and unconnected pieces of information. These connections open the door to more possibilities. You can feel free to make any association you wish without worrying whether others will understand you. An entrepreneur looking for new products mapped out various ideas. The map reminded him of analysis, which reminded him of psychotherapy, which reminded him of Sigmund Freud. He wrote "Sigmund Freud" and drew a bubble around it. The bubble reminded him of a pillow, and that association inspired his idea. He's manufacturing a pillow with Freud's picture on it and marketing it as a tool for do-it-yourself analysis.

4. *Clustering.* The map's organization comes close to the way in which your mind clusters concepts, which makes the mapped information more accessible to the brain. Once your ideas are clustered, try to adopt the viewpoint of a critic seeing the ideas for the first time. This process allows you to test your associations, spot missing information, and pinpoint areas in which you need more and better ideas. Mind mapping is an idea generator. It does not supply raw material, so your map may show areas in which you need to collect more information.

For an example of this technique, look at the process of knitting as completed by mind mapping with bubbles as shown in the student sample map of knitting (see Worksheet 6-5B).

Wallas considered creativity to be a legacy of the evolutionary process that allowed humans to quickly adapt to rapidly changing environments. The assumption behind his model is that creative thinking is a subconscious process that cannot be directed and that creative and analytical thinking are complementary (Wallas, 1926). That being the case, Worksheets 6-4 and 6-5 should serve to facilitate your creative process using each of the techniques described above. By having you think analytically about a challenging situation, the intent is for you to see how you are able to come up with a creative result or solution.

Unit 3: Using the Language of Occupational Therapy To Think Creatively

This unit will have the student utilize the language of occupational therapy to think creatively. Worksheets incorporating the domain of occupational therapy as represented by the *OTPF* (AOTA, 2008), will be emphasized.

The Language of Occupational Therapy

The *OTPF* (AOTA, 2008) represents the current language of our profession. Now in its second edition, it has evolved over time and experienced several revisions. Starting in 1979 with *Uniform Terminology for Reporting Occupational Therapy Services* (AOTA, 1979), our profession established this standard reporting system intended to be applicable for client documentation, reimbursement, and research. It aimed to serve as a common language to facilitate communication between occupational therapists and occupational therapy assistants, third-party payers, and other health care practitioners and to greatly reduce documentation discrepancies.

During its evolution, the *OTPF* has taken many forms, retaining basic terms, modifying others, and adding new language. It is expected that other documents will emerge as our profession continues to become more sophisticated in its conceptual base and practice approaches. However, regardless of it evolutionary language, learning activity analysis is foundational for all occupational therapy practitioners.

For learning purposes, a diagrammatic representation of the *OTPF*, incorporating the latest terminology in the domain component of the document, has been created in Appendix A.

Becoming familiar with this language is an essential skill for any occupational therapy student. In this unit, the student is asked to use these terms not only to facilitate analysis of an activity but also to take it one step further and think in a creative mode. For example, bathing is a basic activity of daily living (ADL) and can be analyzed as it is typically done. However, given the case of a client experiencing moderate-stage Alzheimer's disease who refuses to bathe per the request of the caregiver, a new solution, creatively fashioned by the practitioner in collaboration with the caregiver, is necessary for successful occupational performance to occur.

Analyzing Occupational Performance Creatively

Worksheet 6-6 provides the student with an opportunity to practice analyzing occupational performance and to hone the skill of creating innovative solutions for a specific client profile.

Unit 4: Applying Creativity to Client Intervention

Using case studies and illustrative examples, the student will problem solve for ways in which creative interventions can be designed for therapeutic application. Consequently, the student will be able to develop creative therapeutic interventions for a variety of adults of different ages.

In this portion of the learning process, the student is being asked to create an intervention plan that is innovative, original, and untested in previous scenarios. That may seem like a risky proposition for an entry-level student. However, the following case studies are meant to challenge the student to think outside of the box, or at least to think about what is in the box and how it can be opened to reveal the creative potential in the intervention and in the client.

According to Michalko (2006), "everything new is just an addition or modification to something that already existed" (p. 72). A method that he describes in his book *Thinkertoys* is called *SCAMPER*, which is a mnemonic for a checklist of idea-generating questions developed from Alex Osborn, a pioneer teacher of creativity, and later arranged by Bob Eberle (p. 74).

Substitute something.

Combine it with something else.

Adapt something to it.

Modify or **M**agnify it.

Put it to some other use.

Eliminate something.

Reverse or **R**earrange it.

This method stimulates your thinking into taking alternative pathways of conceptualizing an idea into diverse directions. These nine techniques can transform an object or process into something new. Michalko provides the example of a paper clip and how a manufacturer improved his product by asking the following questions (p. 75):

Identify and describe the "situation": _____

- What can be *substituted* in the clip?
- What can I *combine* the clip with to make something else?
- What can I *adapt* to the clip?
- How can I *modify* the clip?
- What can I *magnify* or add to the clip?
- What *other uses* can I find for the clip?
- What can be *eliminated* from the clip?
- What is the *reverse* of clipping?
- What *rearrangement* of the clip might be better?

Color-coded plastic clips were the result!

As you read and work through the case studies of young, middle-aged, and older adults, apply these techniques to stimulate your problem-solving and clinical reasoning skills so that the outcome is a therapeutic and creative intervention plan. Use Worksheet 6-7 to complete this assignment; see Worksheet 6-8 for a description of case studies of clients in young adulthood (case 1), middle adulthood (case 2), and older adulthood (case 3).

CONCLUSION

In this chapter, several approaches to applying creativity in practice have been explained, and opportunities to develop treatment planning skills have been provided. Experiences of building upon existing skills to analyze activities, incorporating the occupational therapy process and domains in treatment planning, and creatively exploring and designing specific interventions were given in case study scenarios.

As a closing exercise, reflect upon what you have discovered in yourself while completing these worksheets, and answer the following questions.

QUESTIONS

1. How would you describe what it was like for you to tap into your creative potential? What did you learn about yourself in the process?

2. When thinking about a challenging task now, how will you approach it differently than before this learning experience?

3. How might you develop and infuse creativity into a client intervention plan? What factors will you consider, and what steps will you take?

REFERENCES

American Occupational Therapy Association. (1979). *Uniform terminology for reporting occupational therapy services.* Rockville, MD: American Occupational Therapy Association.

American Occupational Therapy Association. (2008). Occupational therapy practice framework: Domain and process (2nd ed.) *American Journal of Occupational Therapy, 62,* 625-683.

Carroll, L. (2005, 1865) *Alice's adventures in wonderland.* New York, NY: Sterling.

Fromm, E. (1959). The creative attitude. In H. Anderson, ed. *Creativity and its cultivation.* London: Harper and Row.

Griffiths, S. & Corr, S. (2007). The use of creative activities with people with mental health problems: A survey of occupational therapists. *British Journal of Occupational Therapy, 70*(3), 107-114.

Michalko, M. (2006) *Thinkertoys: A handbook of creative-thinking techniques* (2nd ed.). Berkeley, CA: Ten Speed Press.

Perrin, T. (2001). Don't despise the fluffy bunny: A reflection from practice. *British Journal of Occupational Therapy, 64*(3), 129-134.

Schmid, T. (2005). *Promoting health through creativity: For professionals in health, arts and education.* London, UK: Whurr Publishers.

Wallas, G. (1926) *The art of thought.* London: Jonathan Cape.

SUGGESTED READINGS

Cropley, A. J. (2001). *Creativity in education and learning: A guide for teachers and educators.* London, UK: RoutledgeFalmer.

Griffiths, S. (2008). The experience of creative activity as a treatment medium. *Journal of Mental Health, 17*(1), 49-63.

Hersch, G. I., Lamport, N. K., & Coffey, M. S. (2005). *Activity analysis: Application to occupation* (5th ed.). Thorofare, NJ: SLACK Incorporated.

Kuhaneck, H. M., Spitzer, S. L., & Miller, E. (2010) *Activity analysis, creativity and playfulness in pediatric occupational therapy: Making play just right.* London, UK: Jones & Bartlett Learning

Murray, C. (2010). Fostering student creativity. *OT Practice, 15*(17), 9-12.

Pierce, D. E. (2003). *Occupation by design: Building therapeutic power.* Philadelphia, PA: F. A. Davis.

Sternberg, R. J., & Williams, W. M. (1996). *How to develop student creativity.* Alexandria, VA: Association for Supervision and Curriculum Development.

Straker, D. (1997). *Rapid problem solving with post-it notes.* Aldershot, UK: Gower.

Worksheet 6-1

Article Critique

The student will search for, summarize, and write a critique of two articles that describe creativity being used by occupational therapy practitioners. A list of suggested resources is provided in Appendix D.

Everyone is expected to read the article by Griffiths and Corr (2007), which provides a brief synopsis of the historical use of creative activities in occupational therapy. References may be extracted from this article. For the written critique (two to three pages in length, double spaced, 11-point font), you should do the following:

- Provide a citation of the article.
- Write a brief summary (highlight the major points and describe your understanding of the "message" of the article).
- Explain how creativity is described/defined.
- Describe how creativity is demonstrated/illustrated, and provide an example.
- Offer the implications for occupational therapy or how the concepts presented could be implemented in therapy.
- In one sentence, state what lasting impression you will take from this article.

Worksheet 6-2

Analyzing Your Creative Potential: Creativity Awareness Form

Think about a time when you had to solve a problem, develop a solution to a question or puzzling situation, and/or face a new challenge, and respond to the following:

1. Identify the situation.

2. Describe the situation in 10 sentences or less.

3. How did you go about solving the question or developing a solution (i.e., what was your thinking process at that time)? What feelings did you express?

4. Is this your usual pattern, or did you have to come up with a new response?

5. Did the situation have a satisfying outcome? If so, how? If not, what were some of the barriers?

6. If faced with a similar situation, would you approach it differently now? If so, how?

7. Detail what you think were the creative components that contributed to your solution.

Worksheet 6-3

Journaling Your Creativity

Create a journal, which you will use for the entire course, to document how you approached a puzzling and/or new situation (either personal or academic), the response you made (novel or routine), and your satisfaction with the outcome. One entry per week should get you moving along with this process. At various points throughout the course, the instructor may ask you to bring the journal to class and share some of your stories. The following is a template for your journal, but you may modify it to fit your creativity (as long as the requested information is included).

Entry: _____   Date: _____

Identify the situation:

Describe the process:

Worksheet 6-4

Applying the Wallas Model

Using the five-stage model of creative thought, analyze a time when you were confronted with a situation that was problematic or had no automatic answer but you were able to come up with a solution.

1. Preparation

   How did you focus on the problem at hand?

   How did you prepare for problem resolution?

   What were the problem's dimensions or characteristics?

   Were there any ethical issues?

2. Incubation

   How long were you unaware of the problem?

   Were there moments of going to and fro thinking of the problem?

   Did you sense that nothing was happening externally?

3. Intimation

    Were you feeling like a solution was on its way?

    How so?

4. Illumination/Insight

    How did the creative idea/solution become apparent to you?

    When did you find yourself aware of the idea?

5. Verification

    How was the idea verified and/or confirmed?

    What were you feeling/thinking when the idea became "real?"

    How was the idea applied?

    What were you thinking then?

Worksheet 6-5

Activity Analysis of a Challenging Task

After experimenting with mapping and think bubbles using your own ideas and separate thoughts, use the following form to analyze your results:

1. Identify the task.

2. Describe the challenge in two to three sentences.

3. Refer to the *OTPF* graphic (see Appendix A), and analyze the task according to the following components:
   a. What is the area of occupation?

   b. What performance skills are being used?
      ○ Sensory perceptual

      ○ Motor

      ○ Emotional

      ○ Cognitive

      ○ Social

c. Are values/beliefs/spirituality inherent in the task?

d. What performance patterns are being used?

e. How is the context influencing the task?

f. What are the primary activity demands of the task?

4. List any other observations about the task that emerged from the analysis.

Now, compare your responses with those of a partner, discuss each other's maps, bubbles, and analyses, and ask each other the following reflective questions:

- What did you learn from this activity?

- What did you learn from your partner?

- What will you do differently the next time you are confronted with a challenging task?

Student Sample 1

Activity Analysis of a Challenging Task (Student Example, Knitting)

1. Identify the task.

   This activity consists of knitting a scarf using knitting needles and yarn.

2. Describe the challenge in two to three sentences:

   The challenge of this activity is that I have never done it before! And, I'm feeling a bit anxious about learning the most basic stitch and even how to begin. The scarf is for myself so when I do make mistakes, I'll be the one who will have to wear it or just store it away!

3. Refer to the *OTPF* graphic (see Appendix A), and analyze the task according to the following components:

   a. What is the area of occupation?

   The area of occupation is leisure participation.

   b. What performance skills are being used?

   ○ Sensory perceptual

   Several skills are in play here, including: locate the tools and yarn; respond to the feel of the yarn; organize the materials; remember the look and feel of the stitches; visual action for sure; proprioceptive and tactile skills are continually being called upon; having to position my body in an upright sitting position; and locate by touch the yarn and needles.

   ○ Motor

   Having to move and physically interact with materials and tools, in contact with objects, locating myself in an environment conducive to learning a new task, reach for yarn, pace myself, coordinate my movements (especially bilateral coordination), anticipate and adjust the pattern and stitches, and manipulate the tools.

   ○ Emotional

   I need to manage my time and feelings of frustration. Through this activity, I'm expressing creativity by color and pattern. I persist to complete the task and as I learn the stitches, I am feeling more in control.

   ○ Cognitive

   I had to plan what would be created, decide on a pattern, at the end judge whether my work was up to expectations, definitely sequence the stitches so they make the pattern, and create what I think will be an attractive product.

   ○ Social

   This knitting task could be done alone or in the company of others. If in a group or with an instructor, I would then need to communicate and interact with them, maintain my physical space, possibly initiate and answer questions, and acknowledge another person's perspective about knitting as a leisure activity and the appeal of the end product.

   c. Are values/beliefs/spirituality inherent in the task?

   Yes, in that I value this activity as a beneficial leisure occupation and have a belief in myself to complete the task and have an attractive end product.

   d. What performance patterns are being used?

   The routine of coming back to this leisure occupation implies satisfaction and serves my roles as friend (perhaps learning the task from a friend or, once proficient in the task, giving it as a gift to a friend), amateur hobbyist, and student, if being taught the stitches.

e. How is the context influencing the task?

The context can have a great influence while performing this task. For example, culturally, there are expectations and creative opportunities; physically, I'm working with objects and tools; socially, I could perform this activity in a group; personally, my age and developmental and economic status are appropriate for this task; meaning is derived from a completed product; temporally, I perform this task at a time of day when I may want to relax; and virtually, I can obtain directions from the Internet.

f. What are the primary activity demands of the task?

The primary activity demands of knitting are dealing with tools and materials (needled and yarn); having the physical space, lighting, and low level of noise that facilitate successful performance; definitely following a sequence of stitches to form a pattern; having intact body functions and structures and performance skills is required to complete this task.

4. List any other observations about the task that emerged from the analysis.

It was satisfying to complete the knitting task and manage the challenge of learning a new leisure activity. I may just do it again!

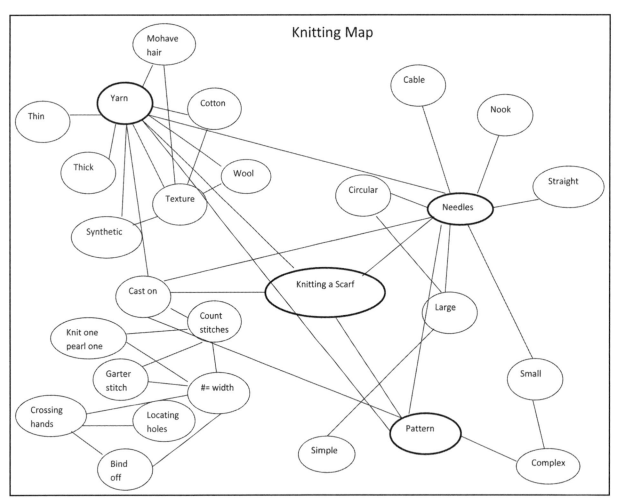

Student sample of "mapping" using knitting as the task. (Reprinted with permission from Cissette Muster, MOT.)

Student Sample 2

Activity Analysis of a Challenging Task (Student Example, Game)

Our Creative Process: Wheel of Rehab Game, Created by Alisha Romero and Marisa Barra, Spring 2012

When given the assignment to come up with a way of teaching the class the topic of rehabilitation with the older adult population for fieldwork seminar, we were instructed to make it interactive. Our professor mentioned that game show-based presentations were done in the past. As soon as we heard the words "interactive" and "game," our wheels were spinning.

We immediately knew that we wanted a game that:

1. Encouraged movement and energy

2. Offered a variety of opportunities for points, because every student differs on the type of question he or she is best at answering

3. Pushed for teamwork, anticipation, and encouragement of others

4. Could be related to the older adult population

5. Would be an enjoyable way to learn and review important information

From these original ideas, we simply began brainstorming ways to accomplish out goals. This thought process was nonlinear. We jumped from idea to idea, utilized trial-and-error problem solving, and attempted to consider all the possibilities of how the game would work without an audience because we are quite familiar with our classmates' dynamic. It is not easy to put our creative process into step-by-step progressive sentences, because the process is not linear or even organized at all times.

The best way to describe it is by providing examples of some of our brainstorming questions and thoughts:

What is a familiar game we can use besides Jeopardy?

- Family Feud
  - How will we determine what the survey says is the most common answer?
  - Ask our classmates? Is that a little too much work? We can only choose multiple-answer questions.
  - We don't want them to stay sitting; what can we do to make them stand up at each turn?
- 2 people stand up then hit a bell to answer
  - But maybe that becomes a matter of who is faster and not who knows the answer.
  - It's been done before.
- Each person comes up and spins the wheel for Wheel of Fortune
  - Where do we get a wheel?
    - We can make one or borrow the one from student life that I have seen before.
    - Perfect, we will ask to borrow it!
- Now that we have the wheel, how many spaces, and what do we put in it?
  - There are 12 spaces. We want different types of questions so it can be more interesting and of varying levels.
  - Well, we can do multiple choice, true of false, or fill in the blank.
    - Some are easier than others.
    - Well, we can make the points different for each type of question, with the easiest being worth fewer points.

- We need something that mimics the vacations for bonus money on Wheel of Fortune.

  - We can double points, lose a turn, or use bankrupt.

  - Lose a turn and bankrupt might be too discouraging; double points it is.

  - But, to get the double points, they have to do an activity to get up and move! Let's make it fun, add music, and relate it to the older adult population. For example, "you are teaching a line-dancing class at the community center; practice your YMCA moves."

- It is so quiet in the class, how can we encourage them to support their teammates and get excited when they get an answer right?

  - We can ask that they clap when the wheel is spinning, like on the show Wheel of Fortune.

  - That will keep them involved when it is not their turn.

  - We can also make noisemakers to shake when their teammate gets the answer right!

  - Perfect! We can use beans in a bottle or can.

- How do we put all these different questions on the PowerPoint presentation?

  - We can use hyperlinks within PowerPoint where you have one homepage with each category, and from there you can click on a question to take you there. From the question slide, you can click the Wheel of Fortune symbol to go back to the home page. The links change colors after they have been used, so we will know not to go back to that question. We can also embed music on the double slides.

Our Product

Wheel of Rehab is an interactive learning game. The game is based on and resembles the popular game show, Wheel of Fortune. While entertaining, the game was also used to integrate information about occupational therapy rehabilitation. The game was chosen because of its popularity and because it offered opportunities to include a variety of categories. To provide familiarity with the learning material, questions were derived from material that was made available to the whole class 5 days earlier. The object of the game is to answer questions that provide information that expands our knowledge of the role of occupational therapy in rehabilitation. The Wheel of Rehab was modified to fit our topic and included the following categories: true/false, multiple choice, fill-in-the-blank, which does not belong, and double (double the points). There was a scoring scale for each category: true/false = 1 point, multiple choice = 2 points, fill-in-the-blank = 3 points, and which does not belong = 2 points, and the double will double the current point total your team has earned. The team with the highest score wins. The double category included physical and mental activities focused around the older adult population, through which we hoped to induce motivation, movement, and meaningful activities, such as flip-flop bean-bag toss, YMCA, circus act (pretend juggling), dancing to "Staying Alive," pretend swimming, word search, Price is Right (shopping), and interaction with teammates. (Further instructions for our activities can be found on the Wheel of Rehab PowerPoint sample slides.)

The supplies that we used included the following:

- A spin wheel borrowed from Student Life
- Construction paper to make the categories for the spin wheel
- Flips the faces (plastic bowls with facial expressions)
- Bean bags
- Beans in water bottles for noisemakers
- Music obtained from the Internet to encourage improvisations and enrich the activities
- Computer to display the PowerPoint slides
- Small dry-erase board for keeping score

The game included two teams of five members each who took turns spinning the wheel. Each team member had to participate in answering questions or doubling their team points. A PowerPoint presentation was used to disperse the questions, music, and activities. Prize bags were given to everyone, because everyone was a winner for participating!

Worksheet 6-6

Analysis of Occupational Performance

Using the form below, analyze the instrumental activities of daily living for making a cup of hot tea, as you would typically do it.

1. Identify the 10 major steps needed to accomplish this activity.

   ○ What key performance skills (motor, praxis, sensory-perceptual, emotional, cognitive, communication/social) are required?

   ○ How different are your steps from those of other students? How similar?

   ○ In class, during small-group discussion, compare your analysis with those of other students.

2. Using the same form and the same activity of making a cup of hot tea, brainstorm with your small group the ways in which you would have a 75-year-old woman diagnosed with early- to moderate-stage Alzheimer's disease perform the same task where she currently resides, in her daughter's home. Making a cup of tea was an important and meaningful task that she performed for herself when she lived alone.

As an added bonus class activity, role-play with another student the intervention session that you would conduct with this client, incorporating the prescribed sequence of steps and components.

Activity Summary and Areas of Occupation

Student Name: _____   Date: _____

Activity: _____

Using the selected activity, provide the information needed to describe it in the categories listed below.

Section A: Activity Description

1. Activity (include name and a brief two- to three-sentence description)

2. Activity demands

   A. *Objects and their properties*

      1. Tools and equipment (nonexpendable)

      2. Materials/supplies (expendable)

   B. *Space demands*, including the specific arrangement of furniture, placement of equipment and supplies, lighting (direct, overhead, task) and ventilation needs (air conditioning, air intake, room temperature), level of acceptable noise/distractions under which the activity can be performed normally.

   C. *Social demands* required to perform the activity, including the involvement of other people, their relationship and expectations of each other (helper, as needed, or for supervision), typical rules, norms, and expectations involved in doing this activity (such as sharing supplies, quiet conversation, exchanging ideas and advice).

   D. *Sequence and timing* of each step, including the specific amount of time required to complete each step and the time required between steps, such as waiting for paint to dry or food to thaw, and the overall time needed for completion of the activity; when the activity would typically be performed (season, time of day, day of the week).

   E. *Precautions*, including the potential safety or health hazards of performing this activity as you plan to do.

   F. *Acceptable criteria* for the completed activity.

Section B: Areas of Occupation

1. Area of occupation: Consider which primary category(ies) the activity would most likely be placed under in the *OTPF* and list it (them) here.

2. Relationship to other areas of occupation: Note performance skills from the *OTPF* that are enhanced by doing this activity (i.e., prepare for, overlap with, or are carried over into other activities in other occupational areas).

   A. Consider which other areas of occupation may be addressed in conjunction with performing the activity, and list them here.

   B. Consider if this activity could be a prerequisite to performing other areas of occupation, and list them here.

   C. Consider what other areas of occupation could be a prerequisite to performing the activity, and list them here.

Section C: Client Factors and Performance Skills

Select only those areas that apply to the activity as it is typically performed. When you analyze it according to a specific case scenario, imagine how it might be different from your performance (e.g., in length of time, attention, effort, value).

1. Client factors

   A. Values, beliefs, spirituality

   B. Body functions

   C. Body structures

2. Performance skills

   A. Motor and praxis skills

   B. Sensory-perceptual skills

   C. Emotional regulation skills

   D. Cognitive skills

   E. Communication and social skills

Section D: Performance Patterns and Context/Environment

1. Performance patterns

   A. Routines

   B. Rituals

   C. Roles

2. Context/environment

   A. Cultural

   B. Personal

   C. Temporal

   D. Virtual

   E. Physical

   F. Social

Worksheet 6-7

Process of Occupational Therapy: The Client Intervention Plan

1. Evaluation

    A. Client profile

    i. Include age, gender, ethnicity, secondary diagnoses, family living arrangements, social support system, occupational history, current occupational roles, and any other information you think is relevant to understanding the client's background and situation.

    ii. Include current status in the following areas of occupation:

        a. Personal ADL

        b. Instrumental ADL

        c. Work/school

        d. Play/leisure

        e. Social participation

    iii. Identify any issues/problems that interfere/challenge successful occupational engagement and participation.

    iv. What has been done to address these issues/problems? (e.g., what strategies, if any, has the individual and/or family used to address these issues?)

        a. What are the client's priorities and goals?

        b. What is the client willing to do? (i.e., motivation)

        c. Identify the context(s) in which the client performs his or her occupational roles; explain the physical, social, cultural, and spiritual factors that affect those roles.

    B. Analysis of occupational performance

    i. Several resources may be used to analyze the client's occupational performance. You can draw from any of the following: synthesis of the occupational profile; observation; selected assessments.

    ii. From these data, you begin to reason and develop possible hypotheses regarding the client's strengths and limitations.

    iii. Create goals based on the information collected from the profile and analysis, as if in collaboration with the client.

2. Intervention

    A. Develop an intervention plan with an objective and measurable goals.

    B. Identify the type(s) of interventions that you may use, and describe your therapeutic use of occupations and activities.

    i. What activities/occupations will you implement with the client? Explain.

    ii. Specify one activity, and document according to the domain and process only those items that are applicable to this one activity.

    C. Identify the intervention approach you would choose, and provide a rationale for its selection.

    D. What outcomes are most appropriate for this client? How will you measure the outcome(s)?

Case Study (Student Sample 3)

Presently, Ms. B, an 87-year-old woman living in senior apartment housing, is at a fairly high level of independence and self-sufficiency. Her one-bedroom apartment has the safety features found in subsidized housing that caters to older adults (e.g., emergency pull in the bathroom and grab bars in the shower). She is able to take care of all her personal and instrumental needs; she has received counseling and medication for depression. In past visits, her physician commented on her osteoporosis getting worse and the need for her to take greater care while moving about. She walks with stooped shoulders and a guarded gait and occasionally requires a cane and assistance for outside ambulation. Her only son lives out of state, but she has made many friends in the apartment complex and is presently vice president of the senior group at the community center, where she attends meetings twice a week and receives a hot lunch. Ms. B is an avid reader and enjoys watching news shows and PBS programming. In addition, she babysits weekly for a 7-year-old boy who enjoys learning from her and playing highly competitive Scrabble games with her. Because of her close-knit relationship with the family of this boy, she has given them several pieces of her favorite china.

Recently, on a wintry morning when leaving the apartment complex, she fell on a patch of ice and fractured her forearm and bruised herself quite badly. The apartment manager spotted her on the ground and called for help. Ms. B was hospitalized for a few days after her forearm was surgically stabilized (closed reduction of the distal radius) and placed in a plaster cast. Frequent complications she suffers are stiffness of her fingers and shoulder and swelling. Cast immobilization usually lasts for 3 to 8 weeks. In order for Ms. B to return home, certain supportive alternatives were arranged, including homemaker assistance and therapy through a home health agency.

1. Evaluation

   A. Client profile

      i. Include age, gender, ethnicity, secondary diagnoses, family living arrangements, social support system, occupational history, current occupational roles and any other information you think is relevant to understanding the client's background and situation.

         Ms. B is an 87-year-old woman who lives in a senior residential apartment with safety features. Before admission, she was independent in all ADL, except she occasionally required a cane and assistance for outside ambulation. She was also fairly active in her community and enjoyed reading, watching television, and the company of a nearby family for whom she babysat. She has a history of depression and osteoporosis. Her current primary diagnosis is a forearm fracture with surgical repair.

      ii. Client's current status in the following areas of occupation: *Not specifically stated in the case, but most areas of occupation will need to be completed with one-handed techniques for the duration of cast immobilization.*

         a. Personal ADL: *Modified independence.*

         b. Instrumental ADL: *Modified independence.*

         c. Work/school: *Modified independence.*

         d. Play/leisure: *Modified independence.*

         e. Social participation: *Independent.*

         Identify any issues/problems that interfere with/challenge successful occupational engagement and participation. *Ms. B needs occasional moderate to minimum assistance with outdoor mobility. In addition, she lives alone, and her son lives in another state.*

      iii. What has been done to address these issues/problems? (e.g., what strategies, if any, has the individual and/or family used to address these issues?) *Ms. B uses a cane for ambulation. She lives in a senior apartment with the usual safety features found in subsidized housing that caters to older adults.*

      iv. What are the client's priorities and goals? *Not specifically stated in the case, but knowing that she was a very independent woman before the accident, it may be assumed that she would want to return to that level of independence.*

v. What is the client willing to do? (i.e. motivation) *Not specifically stated in the case. Again, knowing that she was a very independent woman before the accident, it is likely that she will be motivated to do whatever is needed to be independent. One precaution would be for the therapist to be aware of any signs of depression that could negatively influence her motivation.*

vi. Identify the context(s) in which the client performs his or her occupational roles; explain the physical, social, cultural, and spiritual factors that impact those roles. *Ms. B performs her occupational roles in her senior apartment residence, the community center, and the home where she babysits. She has social supports in the apartment complex and community center. The complications from her surgery of finger and shoulder stiffness and swelling will compromise her participation in various activities. Additionally, her cast immobilization will last anywhere from 3 to 8 weeks, limiting her return to her typical activities, occupational performance, and social participation.*

B. Analysis of occupational performance

i. Several resources may be used to analyze the client's occupational performance. You can draw from any of the following: synthesis of the occupational profile; observation; selected assessments. *As a therapist, you would observe the client as she attempts self-care activities in her home, which provides essential data for planning an intervention plan. In addition, assessments like the Canadian Occupational Performance Measure, range of motion, and an edema measure may contribute vital information for intervention planning.*

ii. From these data, you begin to reason and develop possible hypotheses regarding the client's strengths and limitations. *For example, Ms. B's strengths: previous independence, work ethic, and social engagement; limitations: limited use of upper extremity in performing desired activities, inability to engage in social activities.*

iii. Create goals based on the information collected from the profile and analysis, as if in collaboration with the client. *See the intervention plan.*

2. Intervention

A. Develop an intervention plan with an objective and measurable goals.

Objective: To promote independent occupational participation in self-care activities for her to resume her previous level of function.

Long-term goal: The client will independently complete grooming activities with a one-handed technique in 1 week.

Short-term goal: The client will wash her hair with a one-handed technique with minimum assistance in 2 days.

Short-term goal: The client will brush and/or style her hair with a one-handed technique with minimum assistance in 4 days.

Long-term goal: The client will independently shower with a one-handed technique in 1 week.

Short-term goal: The client will independently demonstrate knowledge of plaster cast precautions and care in 1 day.

Short-term goal: The client will demonstrate transfers into and out of her shower safely with a one-handed technique in 3 days.

B. Identify the type(s) of interventions that you may use, and describe your therapeutic use of occupations and activities.

i. What activities/occupations will you implement with the client? Explain. *Self-care activities will be used with the client, because that is what will be most relevant to Ms. B to reach her previous level of independence.*

ii. Specify one activity, and document according to the domain and process only those items that are applicable to this one activity.

The activity of grooming, specifically hair care, can be analyzed in terms of the following: Client factors—body function due to limitation incurred by cast; performance skills—limited motor and sensory function, pain and discomfort are possible; performance patterns—her usual routine of hair care has been disrupted; contextual factors—personal, temporal, physical, and social components are all impacted by the upper extremity immobility caused by the cast.

C. Identify the intervention approach you would choose, and provide a rationale for its selection. *Modification approach—before admission, Ms. B was mostly independent. Due to her history of depression, it's important that we find ways to compensate for the use of only one arm to enable as much independence as possible.*

D. What outcomes are most appropriate for this client? How will you measure the outcome(s)? *Returning to her previous level of independence is very important for this client. This will be measured by short- and long-term goal achievement as well as any outcome measures that are identified as assessments/measures during the evaluation phase of treatment.*

Worksheet 6-8

Cases for Applying the Client Intervention Plan

Young Adulthood (Ages 21 to 40)

1. Mental retardation: 35-year-old woman who lives in a group home; because of her short attention span and hyperactivity, she is annoying to other clients

2. Bipolar disorder with manic episodes: 30-year-old woman; homemaker and mother of two preschool-aged children; few vocational skills

3. Multiple sclerosis: 40-year-old woman with incoordination of her upper extremities; easily fatigued, even when dressing

4. Below-knee amputation resulting from an industrial accident: 25-year-old single man; wants to return to previous work in the same automotive factory

5. Depression with self-destructive ideation: 25-year-old single woman; secretary; has her own apartment and two cats

6. Closed head injury due to automobile accident: 25-year-old man with mild confusion and occasional emotional outbursts; family includes wife and infant; works as a newspaper artist at home in a corner of his bedroom

7. Second-degree burns: 26-year-old man burned on face, chest, and forearms; now in a rehabilitation unit; mail carrier

8. Guillain-Barré syndrome: 31-year-old woman with limited upper extremity strength and endurance; married, no children; owns a floral shop with her husband; goes to work in the mornings; tires easily but maintains office duties

9. Paraplegia (T10/T11): 34-year-old man; truck driver; wants to return to long-haul driving

10. Chronic schizophrenia: 35-year-old woman with poor academic and social skills; low frustration tolerance

11. Carpal tunnel syndrome: 35-year-old piano accompanist; homemaker, two school-aged children

12. Lung cancer, arrested: 35-year-old woman; secretary; married, no children

13. Congenital blindness: 38-year-old man; basket maker; part of a family crafts business; needs to learn business skills to handle his firm's financial affairs

Middle Adulthood (Ages 41 to 65)

1. Left cerebral vascular accident, right-sided hemiplegia with expressive aphasia: 52-year-old man; civil engineer; married, two teenaged children; lives at home

2. Mid-stage Parkinson's disease: 60-year-old man; widower; retired railroad engineer; lives in an extended care unit of a local retirement community

3. Myocardial infarction: 50-year-old man; family includes wife and three school-aged children; workaholic businessman with few leisure interests

4. Right cerebral vascular accident, left-sided hemiparesis: 65-year-old woman with short attention span and poor spatial judgment with resulting dressing apraxia

5. Hand injury due to an industrial accident: 45-year-old man with poor grasp and weak pronation; plans to return to his job as a dock supervisor

6. Terminal breast cancer: 55-year-old woman; married, two grown children; former bank teller; interested in quilting; receives hospice care at home

7. Rheumatoid arthritis with involvement of wrists and hands: 56-year-old woman; widow and recently retired schoolteacher

8. Rheumatoid arthritis: 42-year-old woman; homemaker, four school-aged children

9. Emphysema: 57-year-old businessman; married; preparing for retirement

Older Adulthood (Ages 66 and older)

1. Parkinson's disease: 78-year-old woman; lives in a long-term care facility; widow with one daughter who lives in an adjoining state; uses a walker for ambulation; tires easily

2. Mid- to late-stage Alzheimer's disease: 80-year-old woman; lives in a nursing home; husband visits her daily

3. Late-onset diabetes: 68-year-old woman; has four grown children living in the same city; wants to continue living in her own home

4. Right hip fracture: 75-year-old woman; in skilled care facility for 10 days; rehabilitation emphasis is on daily life skills before being discharged to home; married, husband at home but frail

5. Left cerebral vascular accident with resulting right-sided hemiparesis: 70-year-old woman; lives alone; hopes to return to her apartment on the second floor (no elevator)

Benefits of Creativity:
Building Professional Skills

Defining/identifying creativity

Recognizing/acknowledging use of creativity in OT

Describing the cognitive process of creativity

Understanding the neuroscience and structures of creativity

Incorporating creativity into professional skills

Applying creativity in client intervention

Applying research in creativity

7

Implications of Creativity in Occupational Therapy Research

Tina Fletcher, EdD, MFA, OTR

Although occupational therapy is regarded as a creative health care profession, a clear picture of the role that creativity plays in contemporary occupational therapy practice has been elusive. Understandings of creativity have changed as more about human personality and society has been learned, and new technology has dramatically expanded the ways of conducting research. Occupational therapist researchers Cusick and McCluskey (2000) proposed that occupational therapy practitioners need to reconsider how they feel about using research to guide their clinical reasoning. The amount of creativity research is steadily increasing. Contributions to evidence-based practice can be made by exploring the impact that creativity has on both occupational therapy practitioners and the practice of occupational therapy.

Armed with new knowledge and technology, creativity can be easier than ever to measure, but only if the research questions about creativity and its role in occupational therapy practice are carefully formulated to determine exactly what knowledge is being sought. Collecting creativity information and data can be interesting and often fun, but the preliminary work of designing creativity research can be a great challenge.

From a researcher's perspective, creativity is a complicated matter. In the literature, it is defined in so many ways that it brings to mind the old story of blind men describing an elephant based on what they feel. Like

the differences between an elephant's tail, trunk, and ears, definitions of creativity depend on how it is seen. Creativity can be described as a personal trait or a feeling that a person or group has, or it can describe an object or the environment. In 2008, Furnham and Bachtiar found that there were more than 60 definitions of creativity in the research literature, and the list continues to grow.

Before any research or measurement can begin, a working definition of creativity must be formulated. From its roots in the early 1950s, creativity research has changed continually. Consequently, defining such a rapidly changing concept has been a challenge. A brief review of creativity-related research will show how understanding of creativity have grown like rings on a target. Originally, creativity was seen as a simple personal trait. Over time, rings formed around this bullseye until a much more complex and component-based picture emerged. A creativity researcher's job is to sort through these rings until he or she finds which of them will provide the most help in answering the questions being asked.

This chapter focuses on preliminary research of occupational therapy practitioners' creativity and how they use it to better serve their clients. After a brief review of the creativity literature, the Four P Model of creativity, which examines components of the creative person, process, press (environment), and products in occupational

Coffey MS, Lamport NK, Hersch GI.
Creative Engagement in Occupation: Building Professional Skills (pp 99-108).
© 2015 SLACK Incorporated.

therapy, is discussed. The words of occupational therapy practitioners of different ages and levels of professional experience and from different practice areas illustrate how the creativity experienced in each of these components affects their practice of occupational therapy.

This chapter concludes with considerations about conducting creativity research with human subjects and a brief review of qualitative and quantitative research, and information on how to select creativity-related assessments is presented. Perhaps most importantly, this chapter reinforces the need for us to encourage occupational therapy practitioners and students to consider the role that creativity plays in their own practice and clinical reasoning.

OBJECTIVES

1. Explore the history of creativity research over the past six decades.

2. Distinguish the differences between product-based and process-oriented creativity theories.

3. Identify the outcomes that can be learned by measuring creativity.

4. Explain the Four P Model as it applies to creativity in occupational therapy.

5. Describe each of the four P's (personal, process, press, and product).

6. Provide examples of the Four P Model from occupational therapy practice.

7. Describe considerations to be made when deciding on qualitative or quantitative methods.

8. Compare the outcomes of each method.

9. Explain the ways to evaluate creative products.

UNIT 1: THEORETICAL MODELS OF CREATIVITY

This unit examines creativity research and theories and considers how they have changed over time.

Creativity in the 1950s: Personal Traits

The study of creativity, although relatively new in relation to many other human studies, has been around since former American Psychological Association President J. P. Guilford (1950) charged his colleagues to begin creativity research in earnest. As a reflection of his own interests in applying newly developed modern scientific methods to the study of the seemingly indescribable human mind, Guilford developed the well-regarded Structure of Intellect model of human intelligence. This model conceptualized an individual's intelligence as a series of 150 operations, contents, and products; each was represented as an individual cube, and they all contributed to a large, neat block. The configuration of an individual's cubes was thought to reveal many things about his or her intellectual abilities, including degree of creativity. Although it may seem like a peculiar oversimplification of human intelligence to our modern eyes, Guilford's model, among other things, was used by the United States government to determine the work assignments of men and women who served in the armed forces from the 1950s through the 1970s (Guilford & Hoepfner, 1971).

For many years, subsequent research continued to extend Guilford's assumptions that creativity was a manifestation of an individual's unique intellectual functioning. As a result, researchers believed that the way an individual expressed creativity did not vary with regard to the task at hand, the influence of others, or even the individual's motivations to engage in creative activity. Theoretically, a person's degree of creativity would remain consistent regardless of whether he or she lived and worked in the complete isolation of an Antarctic weather station or with fellow artists in the heart of New York City's teeming SoHo district.

The most notable extension and clarification of this type of personality-based creativity research was in the work of Paul Torrance, who dramatically expanded the field of pencil-and-paper creativity testing. One of Torrance's most important contributions to contemporary understanding of creativity was to note that creativity and intelligence are not always paired; he found that not all highly intelligent people are creative and that not all highly creative individuals are markedly intelligent (Torrance & White, 1969).

Over the years, Torrance conducted numerous rigorous, systematic studies to develop creativity test protocols, and many readers may remember participating in mysterious drawing tests during their elementary school years. Often, those exercises were variations of Torrance's popular test of creative thinking, which measures an amalgam of the attributes of originality, flexibility, novelty, and elaboration. In fact, nearly 40 years after its development, the Torrance Test of Creative Thinking (Torrance, 1966) is still used across the world to determine student placement in gifted-child programs. Likewise, the Torrance Center for Creative Thinking, operated under the auspices of the University of Georgia, continues to serve as a clearinghouse for worldwide creativity research.

Creativity in the 1960s and 1970s: What Surrounds the Person

Despite the fact that the number of paper-and-pencil assessments designed to measure creative personal attributes grew through the 1960s and 1970s, some psychologists began to question whether they were truly valid measures of a person's creativity. They also suggested that the personal traits associated with creative thinking were not as stable over time as early creativity researchers had concluded. Notably, B. F. Skinner, the famous "black-box" psychologist who championed operant conditioning, proposed that, like other behaviors, human creativity was highly influenced by many variables (Catania & Harnad, 1988), and humanist Abraham Maslow (1970) postulated that humans need to have their basic needs of survival and safety met before they can be creative. Likewise, renowned client-centered counselor Carl Rogers (1961) insisted that creativity sprang from an environment characterized by unconditional acceptance and support. Although they differed from each other in some ways, each of these influential theorists shared the belief that creativity resulted from the interaction of personal and social phenomena. In this way, the first ring around the creativity research bullseye was formed.

Creativity in the 1980s and 1990s: Inner States and Outer Recognitions

Building on the contributions of the behavioral humanists from the 1960s and 1970s, a second ring of creativity research formed when happiness and creativity psychologist/researcher Mihaly Csikszentmihalyi (1996) formulated significant new understandings that formalized the role of gatekeepers in creativity. Essentially, Csikszentmihalyi asserted that a process or outcome cannot be considered creative unless the experts from that specific domain recognize it as such. Furthermore, he held to the belief that creative paradigm-shifting "big C" creativity differed from the more commonly seen "little c" creativity, sometimes referred to as *everyday creativity*. Although big C creativity continues to be considered a rare occurrence, little c creativity is viewed as the "building a better mousetrap" type of creativity that everyone experiences to varying degrees. Csikszentmihalyi also conceptualized the phenomenon of creative flow as the experience of pleasurable absorption in a process in which the concept of time and an awareness of one's environment is suspended or altered in some way. During flow, all energies are focused on the creative process itself. In fact, Csikszentmihalyi pointed out that emotions such as happiness and joy really are not part of the flow experience but may follow it in reflection.

Csikszentmihalyi's contributions to understanding creativity are important because they establish a relationship between the inner experiences of flow with the necessary recognition by others that something creative has happened. Recognition by others shows that creativity has relevance to the world, and even in its simplest forms, it is more than just daydreaming or doodling. Csikszentmihalyi's model of creativity acknowledges the significance of the art critic, the reviewer, the panel of judges, or in a much larger extent, the Nobel Prize committee.

Creativity Research in the New Millennium: Drive and Outcomes

Interestingly, like Guilford in the 1950s, a second notable President of the American Psychological Association has devoted his career to further our understanding of intelligence and creativity. Another significant creativity research ring formed when Robert Sternberg (2003) developed the Triarchic Theory of Intelligence, a synthesis of the analytic, practical, and contextual aspects of intelligence and creativity. Importantly, this model steers away from notions that psychometric testing can truly contribute to a valid understanding of an individual's creativity. Placing emphasis on cognition, Sternberg has emphasized the roles that experience, choice, and wisdom play in creative thinking. Seen in this way, levels of creativity can ebb and flow across a lifespan, changing in response to life roles, events, values, and goals.

Further expanding on these growing understandings of creativity as a social phenomenon, Harvard researcher Theresa Amabile (Amabile, 1983; Amabile, Conti, Coon, Lazenby, & Herron, 1996) proposed yet one more conceptual model of creativity that dovetails with Sternberg's creative cognition model. Amabile's componential model stresses that creativity is built on the following three things: task-relevant skills, general creativity-relevant skills, and the personal motivation to engage in a creative task. This model not only factors in personal traits but also expands on what an individual must bring to the creative plate. The individual must understand the rules of the game and must know how to use the materials at hand, what has already been done with them, and what remains to be done. Most significant is that Amabile's model is the first to state that an individual must be motivated to be creative, and she shares with Sternberg the belief (as seen in his Triarchic model) that creativity is a choice.

Amabile further defined the motivation component of her model by differentiating between intrinsic and extrinsic creativity. Intrinsic or internal motivation, she has asserted, is the key factor for true creativity. Amabile has firmly asserted that when creativity stems from intrinsic or internal motivations (such as interest, curiosity, and intellectual energy) rather than from extrinsic or external motivators (such as payment, prizes, recognition, or respect), the outcomes will be more creative and novel while still remaining relevant to the task at hand. In other words, working for monetary gain, stickers, or promotions may induce an individual's superficial creativity, but true creative performances will not emerge until an individual's behavior stems from a deeper, more substantial form of motivation.

To round out understandings of the relationship between creativity and intrinsic, internal motivation, consideration of the phenomenon of burnout merits notice. Theorists Maslach and Jackson (1981) described *burnout* as a phenomenon characterized by emotional exhaustion, depersonalization, and diminished feelings of personal accomplishment. Typically described as a workplace phenomenon, their model of burnout makes it easier to understand how diminishing motivation can be associated with diminished creativity. Because burnout is often associated with employment, both the Amabile and the Maslach and Jackson models are significant to our understanding of creativity in the workplace. Research on creativity in the workplace has a singular identifying phenomenon: it tends to be product or outcome based. In many ways, this differs significantly from the process-oriented flow creativity that Csikszentmihalyi had described. Accordingly, this new product- and outcome-based creativity research brings up a whole new conundrum for researchers: How can creative outcomes be measured? Obviously, paper-and-pencil personality tests are not good methods for measuring creative products. Accordingly, Amabile and her colleagues (1996) devised a method of product assessment called the *consensual assessment technique* (CAT). This method offers an objective and replicable method of assessing creative products and can be used in a variety of contexts.

Unit 2: Using the Four P Model to Understand Creativity in Occupational Therapy

Unit 1 provided an overview of the ways in which creativity research has evolved from models that focus exclusively on creative personal traits to those that incorporate increasingly complex systems, including the environment, the creative experience, and creative outcomes. The Four P Model is a useful tool for understanding creativity and designing creativity research in occupational therapy practice.

Although numerous variations of "P" models exist, Mark Runco's (2004) model is handily composed of the categories person, press (environment), process, and product. Using this model to group the many research findings about creativity enables a potential researcher to organize and see how concepts of creativity align with their own interests. These categories are flexible in design and often show overlapping constructs.

When using a model to understand a concept, it is important to view the model as a helpful, rather than limiting, tool. In other words, how one group views creativity will differ from that of another, depending on their needs and interests. For example, occupational therapy is a process-oriented profession in which a change in client status or function is often viewed as the desired creative outcome or product. A toothpaste manufacturer, however, would place more emphasis on the creative development of a physical product, such as a new and improved tooth-whitening system. The ways in which these two groups view creativity may be similar in some respects but differ widely in others.

A brief review of the Four P Model reveals how each category contributes to a broader understanding of creativity in occupational therapy. Fletcher (2010) interviewed occupational therapy practitioners whose ages spanned from 25 to 65 years about creativity in relation to their practice of occupational therapy. These occupational therapy practitioners had practiced from 2 to over 30 years in settings ranging from school systems and home health agencies to hospitals and skilled nursing facilities. Consistent with Sternberg's (2003) research findings, age and maturity seemed to play a defining role in each of their widely varying relationships with creativity. After a discussion of Four P Model categories, excerpts from these occupational therapy practitioners illustrate how creativity in each category affected their practice and clinical reasoning.

Personal Creativity in Occupational Therapy

The relationships between creativity, occupational therapy, and personality involve several key elements. What creative things happen when a therapist and client form a relationship? Harkening back to Sternberg's model, the therapist must be able to use his or her specialized knowledge and skills to determine the analytic, practical, and contextual aspects of a client's reason for referral. He or she must also be able to modify the treatment plan when a client's condition and circumstances change. Kalischuk and Thorpe (2002) determined that creative problem solving was important to nurses because it helped them successfully juggle clinical care, patient relationships, and their own educational needs, and Albarran (2004) suggested that creativity leads to more resourceful, innovative patient care. Occupational therapy practitioners may experience similar benefits from creativity in their own work.

The clients also hold special knowledge and skills. They alone understand what their abilities were before they needed occupational therapy, and they have their own beliefs and values. In many circumstances, a client will also hold extensive knowledge of the world in which he or she will live when occupational therapy services are no longer being delivered. Although the primary responsibility of therapists is to provide client-centered care, they also must care for their own needs. Maslach and Jackson (1981) noted that, because much of the work in human service professions is linked to a client's difficulties, interactions with them are frequently laden with anger, embarrassment, fear, and despair and frequently deplete these professionals' emotional reserves, leaving them exhausted and cynical. Research in nursing has shown that creativity can be one way to prevent burnout (Berg, Hansson, & Hallberg, 1994; Sandovich, 2005).

For the occupational therapist, the creative trait of *flexibility*, being able to view something in many different ways, is essential for successful occupational therapy practice. The creative trait of *fluency*, generating a large number ideas or problem solutions, also increases the chance that some good, workable treatment plans will occur. The creative trait of *originality*, producing new or novel ideas, can also be important, as long as the creative ideas are practical and relevant.

In her work, Corrie (a pseudonym), a twenty-something occupational therapy practitioner who worked in a hospital, believed that the creative traits of flexibility ("I always have to be changing") and fluency ("I could use everything that I had") contributed to how her creative personality impacted her work. Closer examination also shows how Sternberg's analytic, practical, and contextual components have been a part of her client-centered clinical reasoning. Describing herself as a creative therapist, Corrie ventured:

> *I'm always trying to think outside of the box. I'm looking at a situation and thinking, "How can I make this better?" I think because I'm in acute care, or because of the constant change, the change in patients, their medical status, mental status, emotional status—it's always changing—so I have to be always changing. So I think creativity comes from the experience of knowing what will work and what doesn't work.*

Ricca (a pseudonym), a county hospital practitioner in her late 30s, discussed how her personal creativity helped her manage some of the difficulties she experienced when working in a fast-paced county hospital environment

and potentially staved off burnout. Describing herself as a creative musician, she observed:

> *At the hospital, you get all the spectrum of emotions. I think there's no way to walk away from that and not have it affect what you're doing outside of here. At home I can play my instrument, and I think what I play is very much dictated by how I'm feeling. It's like, am I going to pull out the Mozart or pull out something slower? I just need to do this, and get it all out, and then I can go on.*

Like their occupational therapist counterparts, patients also experience creativity in occupational therapy. As in the case of other personality traits, personal creativity has a predictable pattern of maturation (Roskos-Ewoldsen, Black, & McCown, 2008). In fact, some researchers believe the middle years of adulthood through old age may be the most creative of all, affirming the need for creative fluent, flexible, and original thinking about everyday challenges and changing circumstances that older people face.

Process Creativity in Occupational Therapy

Process creativity can be a slippery term, because people frequently do not have words to describe what happens to them when they are in the midst of a deeply absorbing creative activity. In fact, Nelson and Rawlings (2009) wrote that, because creativity research had neglected the creative process, they developed the Experience of Creativity Questionnaire. When experiencing creativity, it is sometimes hard to say exactly what is happening. Perhaps this is why Csikszentmihalyi's research and writing on the concept of creative flow remain so enthusiastically received. To use occupational therapy parlance, finding flow is like finding the just-right challenge; the task demands must match the abilities of the person. For occupational therapy practitioners, this means that they must have the knowledge and skills to be effective client care providers. If the task demands are greater than the practitioner can manage, he or she may worry and become anxious. On the other hand, if task demands are well below what the practitioner is capable of, he or she may become bored and anxious. In one study, nine occupational therapy practitioners described the creative process in their work as thinking fluidly, drawing from an internalized repertoire of experiences, and making effective, relevant, and sometimes novel and entertaining treatment plans (Fletcher, 2010). In this way, therapists found the just-right challenges of their work, situating their clinical reasoning in the zone between boredom and the worry and anxiety that can block flow.

Regarding her own experience of the creative process, Carly, a mental health practitioner in her 50s, recalled:

> *I love coming up with alternative ideas and solutions. I mean, people have the same diagnosis, but there's something different or unique to them, and you have to really think of it. To me, creativity at work is addressing each individual person and coming up with what motivates them, coming up with activities that you would collaborate on, and that would be meaningful. I call it being able to tap dance.*

Press (Environmental) Creativity in Occupational Therapy

Research exploring creative environments is a relative newcomer to the field of creativity. In fact, Amabile noted that although little has been published on the topic, considerable folklore surrounds creativity that springs from exotic, faraway environments (Amabile et al., 1996). Images of the French artist Paul Gauguin painting Tahitian beauties may come to mind, as might lesser-known anecdotes such as the case of Friedrich Schiller, who reportedly kept apples in his desk because he believed that their smell got his creative juices flowing, especially when they were rotten.

As noted, although early creativity research zeroed in on personality factors, it has been conducted more recently in the workplace. When considering environmental creativity in occupational therapy, there are some unique considerations, because a client receiving occupational therapy services may face a doubled environmental challenge of being treated in a workplace or hospital environment while residing in another. Many considerations relevant to occupational therapy settings echo the findings of Amabile et al. (1996) on environment and creativity: That more creative learning happens when traditional settings are left behind, and both work and home environments without intrusive control are more creative than those run with interfering, autocratic leadership styles. Likewise, playful work and home environments stimulate creativity, and highly competitive or stressful ones do not. So, it seems that key environmental elements known to stimulate creativity include personal freedom, good management, adequate resources and time, nonintrusive but encouraging leadership, recognition, and manageable amounts of challenge.

Fletcher (2010) observed that occupational therapy practitioners tended to be progressively less influenced by some environmental factors as they matured both personally and professionally. With the increasing internal resources of knowledge, skills, and confidence, there is a diminished reliance on external resources, such as supplies, budgets, physical comforts, and the presence of others.

As an example, consider the differences in the way novice and experienced occupational therapy practitioners approached the typical rules and resources associated with cooking. Lynette (a pseudonym), a recently graduated occupational therapy practitioner in her mid-20s, felt that her rule-bound work environment restricted her creativity, while at home she was free to bend some of the rules, which freed her creativity. She said:

> *When I cook, I try to come up with different tastes. I think I enjoy being creative, personally, because I am not under pressure. If I don't have the proper ingredients, I can substitute in cooking; I have to work with what I have. But at work, there is the pressure; we have to learn so many techniques and also to use what we have.*

These thoughts differ from those of Beatrice (a pseudonym), a well-seasoned community-based practitioner in her 60s. While Lynette was trying to learn the ropes, Beatrice had already done so. Unlike Lynnette, she preferred to steer away from recipes and rule-bound areas when cooking:

> *I don't generally think of myself as a creative person by artistic standpoints, but I think being creative is being uniquely yourself, or different from some of the norms: then that would be me. You know, I don't like to follow recipes, and that's why I don't bake well: You have to follow a recipe exactly. In a meal I make entrees, and if I don't have certain ingredients, I think, well, this will do just as well [laughs]. I like that part, but I don't like creating pastries, because you have to do it exactly right.*

Chatalaine (a pseudonym), a skilled nursing facility practitioner in her 50s, showed that like Beatrice, she had learned to navigate many of the challenges of her career and, as a result, did not feel as constrained by environmental circumstances. Instead, she was able to navigate the terrain of rules and regulations and make them work in her favor. She said:

> *Now that I'm older, I've treated in different environments, with different populations, with different kinds of therapists, and with different situations. I feel like I have a stronger foundation of knowing the right buttons to push to be able to be creative and to get the results or the outcomes that I want. You have to have a good foundation, and you have to be self-confident: "I've seen it work with this person, so let me see if it will work here with this patient."*

When Chatalaine was asked if she was creative, she laughed and said:

> *Professionally? Personally? I can be. I can be. If the situation really calls for creativity, I can really whip it out, but I think what's important is responding to our circumstances in our environment; it's*

responding to what our needs are right now. There are times that require us to not be creative, and we have to be very businesslike and straightforward or very functional, and other times in our lives—both professionally and personally—there are times that allow for more creative outlets, and we incorporate some of that into what we do all the time, but there are some times that are better than others.

Another experienced rehabilitation center practitioner, Donna (a pseudonym), echoed her fellow well-seasoned therapists by saying:

> *I've been practicing 25 years. I have seen both ends of the spectrum: new people just out of school [who] aren't as creative because they aren't experienced; they haven't learned as much for their bag of tricks yet, they don't know what to do. But then you've also got the people who have been practicing 20 years [who] are working for different motivations and aren't creative.*

As each of these therapists show, the range of environmental influences on creativity spans factors such as organizational structure, politics, and resources. Research shows that the impact of environmental factors can change over time and with both personal and professional maturation (Fletcher, 2010; Sternberg, 2003).

ACTIVITY 7-1

To understand the potential for creativity in a workplace, complete this questionnaire, and then share your responses with other students.

Rating the Creative Environment

How would you rate your workplace (Mayfield & Mayfield, 2010)?

1. My supervisor encourages me to be creative.

2. My work group is supportive of new ways of doing things.

3. My organization encourages me to work creatively.

4. I have the resources I need to do my job.

5. My work is challenging.

6. I have control over how I do my work.

7. My organization's politics make it difficult to be creative.

8. My organization's policies impede spontaneity in the workplace.

9. It is difficult to be creative with the work deadlines I have.

Product Creativity in Occupational Therapy

As previously discussed, product creativity is a relatively new area of research. One of the challenges has been to measure the degree of creativity in a vast and wide array of products. Clearly, there is no one-size-fits-all method of creative product assessment. Although Taylor and Sandler (1972) devised a Creative Product Inventory and Besemer and O'Quin (1999) made some notable strides with the Creative Product Semantic Scale, there were problems associated with both of these works in relation to language use and measurement validity.

Without question, Amabile et al. (1996) created the most successful method of assessing product creativity to date. The CAT relies on judges who are familiar with the domain of the product or response to evaluate the degree of creativity. The CAT is an objective tool that evaluates the tangible agreed-upon creativity components selected by experts in that field. It is similar to Csikszentmihalyi's (1996) theory, which requires experts from a domain to say whether an individual has been creative. One of the unique aspects of the CAT is that although the degree of creativity is determined by experts, these experts do not have to articulate the reason for their decision. It is ironic that although Amabile et al. insist that only a tangible product or response can be measured by this process, judges are allowed to follow their instincts and use intuition to guide their evaluations. The authors also specified that the judges must operate independently of one another, be experts in the field, and be able to measure other attributes of the products, such as craftsmanship.

It is interesting to note that occupational therapy practitioners report both tangible and intangible things when asked what their creative products are. Young practitioners tend to report physical objects more often, and as practitioners mature professionally, they rely less on the physical and more on the concepts and ideas from their work. For example, Jen (a pseudonym), a school therapist in her 30s, described her creative physical products in the following way:

> *I do a lot of handwriting, so I use a lot of nonslip surfaces. As far as being creative, I would say okay, get them out of the desk, and let them use different writing surfaces. If I'm trying to get a slant or the pencil to lean into the web space, I'll use rubber bands, and I'll put two rubber bands together. So, creativity means if I don't have that specific item, what can I use to improvise?*

Likewise, newcomer Lynette noted:

> *Let's see, just coming up with things like writing paper. If I feel like the ones that they can get from*

a catalogue are not working, I make my own, and then I see what works for the students, like a bunch of writing papers that have graphing lines and a bunch of lines on the paper. I just draw the one or two lines that they need—that kind of creativity—building things [laughs]; I'm actually good at building things.

This contrasts with Chatalaine, the practitioner with more than 30 years of practice under her belt. She described her creative products as follows:

There's loyalty, there's buy in, there's a lot more. I feel like because of my creativity that I am able to inspire other people to do their best, and to make sure that they are advocating and providing the services that are needed for our residents.

Donna, also a well-seasoned practitioner, noted her idea of what a creative product is:

The ultimate creativity would be doing a group activity where you can involve your patient—maybe a party. How can you meet treatment goals, have fun, do something that we both enjoy, outside of the boring what I do every day—and for them too—so the ultimate creativity is to have a party!

Unit 3: Measuring Creativity Using Qualitative and Quantitative Research Methods

Typically, creativity research is performed by using either quantitative or qualitative methods. This unit provides some basic information about each method and emphasizes how they might affect research design decisions.

Selecting Quantitative Methods to Measure Creativity

Using quantitative methods to assess creativity indicates that the researcher seeks to prove or disprove an idea. The research proceeds with a hypothesis that is based on theory. Frequently, statistical analyses of the results of standardized assessments are used to prove or disprove the hypothesis. Many factors exist when considering the right assessment type for gathering data. The following list of considerations explores the decisions that must be made when developing a quantitative research study, selecting the constructs to measure, and choosing measurement tools:

1. What is the research question? What are the research variables?

2. Is the assessment tool based on theory? How reliable and valid is it?

3. Is it possible to locate, afford, and purchase the assessment tool?

4. Does the assessment tool require that the administrator be certified in any way to purchase, use, or interpret it?

5. Is it possible to preview the assessment or to buy a sample? Are discounts available to student researchers?

6. How long does the assessment tool take to administer? Are the results difficult or time-consuming to score? Do scores require outside analysis or special computer capabilities and/or software or have any other special considerations?

7. Is it possible to talk to the test developer or testing company customer service representative to determine if the assessment tool is the best choice for the research design being considered? (They may provide information about other assessments that are new or unfamiliar to the researcher.)

If all of these factors are considered carefully, it is less likely that the reader will end up a hapless consumer when it comes to shopping on the Internet or through testing catalogues or databases for tests. Being prepared can enable an individual to take advantage of the Internet's convenience and still make savvy decisions. Table 7-1 provides information about commonly used quantitative creativity assessments.

Activity 7-2

To see how the Creative Product Semantic Scale (O'Quin & Besemer, 2006) might assess occupational therapy products, think of an occupational therapy product with which you are familiar, such as an orthotic device, an item used in self-care, or a piece of positioning equipment. How would you rate it in the following categories?

- Surprising
- Original
- Logical
- Useful
- Valuable
- Understandable
- Organic

TABLE 7-1. QUANTITATIVE CREATIVITY ASSESSMENTS	
Abbreviated Torrance Test for Adults (Kathy Goff & E. Paul Torrance, 2002)	Creative thinking ability in people over 18 years; fluency, originality, elaboration, and flexibility, with creativity indicators
Creatrix Inventory (Revised) (Richard Byrd & Jacqueline Byrd, 1971-2006)	Person's creative risk-taking propensity, creativity, and risk taking; describes the creative sustainer, modifier, challenger, practicalizer, innovator, synthesizer, dreamer, and planner
Khatena-Torrance Creative Perception Inventory (E. Paul Torrance & Joe Khatena, 1976-1998)	Creative personality and acceptance of authority, self-confidence, inquisitiveness, awareness of others, disciplined imagination, environmental sensitivity, initiative, self-strength, intellectuality, individuality, and artistry
Torrance Tests of Creative Thinking (E. Paul Torrance, 1966-1984)	Creative potential, verbal, figural, fluency, flexibility, originality, elaboration

- Well-crafted

- Elegant

These categories have emerged after 25 years of research into what makes a thing creative. Would you have chosen additional attributes? If so, what are they?

Selecting Qualitative Methods to Measure Creativity

Qualitative data are typically collected by interviewing, watching, analyzing case studies, immersing oneself in a culture, and/or examining archives. In contrast to the research designs of quantitative studies, qualitative studies tend to be more open-ended in terms of what they expect to reveal. Although quantitative studies prove or disprove hypotheses, qualitative studies frequently generate them. Qualitative research requires that an investigator be open to many possibilities, be able to draw conclusions about observations, and be willing to navigate uncertain waters.

Although the qualitative method relies on standardized assessment tools, qualitative methods in creativity research may involve interviewing participants about their creativity, interviewing others about the participant's creativity, taking field notes about things that affect creativity, and documenting and analyzing a product's creativity.

Using the Consensual Assessment Technique to Evaluate Creative Products

Although at first glance the CAT may seem to be a quantitative method of creative product assessment because of its various structures and methods, it is not categorized here as either a quantitative or qualitative methodology. The reader interested in using the CAT should refer to *Creativity in Context* (Amabile, 1996) for specific guidelines. In order for creativity to be assessed by the CAT, the task must have a product or something that can be seen, the task should allow for some flexibility in interpretation, and the task should not be one that depends heavily on specialized skills.

The CAT judges must meet the following criteria: they must be experienced in the domain in question, they must make their assessments independently, and they should also make assessments on dimensions other than creativity, such as technical aspects and aesthetics (to help determine if creativity is related to or independent of those dimensions).

As an example, some categories measured during a fine arts CAT can include creativity, novel use of materials, novel ideas, technical skill, organization, effort, evident planning, and expressiveness.

Final Thoughts

This chapter has introduced readers to the ever-changing field of creativity and creativity research and has discussed how creativity can and does contribute to improved patient outcomes in occupational therapy. Creativity affects every practitioner in his or her personal and professional endeavors, and it changes along with personal maturation and professional experience. Creativity sustains, informs, and entertains. It keeps practitioners engaged in their professional endeavors, surprises them in their personal lives, and sometimes makes them laugh out loud. Studying creativity certainly is worth the effort.

QUESTIONS

1. What effect have the various theories of creativity had on occupational therapy?

2. Describe the Four P Model in your own words; apply it to a creative work you have done.

3. If you were to conduct creativity research, what method appeals to you? Explain your reasoning for that decision.

4. Is it really possible to measure creativity?

5. Given what we know about creativity, what methods are best for measuring it?

6. What do we hope to learn by measuring creativity?

7. Which of the four Ps do you believe is most closely related to creativity?

8. Some experts believe there are even more Ps related to creativity. What do you think they could be?

9. It's hard to imagine that measuring something as fun as creativity would cause problems. What could go wrong, and why?

10. Knowing what you do about research, is creativity measured more accurately by using qualitative methods, quantitative methods, or both?

REFERENCES

Albarran, J. W. (2004). Creativity: An essential element of critical care nursing practice. *Nursing in Critical Care, 9*(2), 47-49.

Amabile, T. M. (1983). The social psychology of creativity: A componential conceptualization. *Journal of Personality and Social Psychology, 45*(2), 357-377.

Amabile, T. M. (1996). *Creativity in context.* Boulder, CO: Westview Press.

Amabile, T. M., Conti, R., Coon, H., Lazenby, J., & Herron M. (1996). Assessing the work environment for creativity. *Academy of Management Journal, 39*(5), 1154-1184.

Berg, A., Hansson, U., & Hallberg, I. R. (1994). Nurses' creativity, tedium and burnout during 1 year of clinical supervision and implementation of individually planned nursing care: Comparisons between a ward for severely demented patients and a similar control ward. *Journal of Advanced Nursing, 20*(4), 742-749.

Besemer, S. P., & O'Quin, K. (1999). Confirming the three-factor creative product analysis matrix model in an American sample. *Creativity Research Journal, 12*(4), 287-297.

Catania, C., & Harnad, S. (Eds.). (1988). *The selection of behavior: The operant behaviorism of B. F. Skinner: Comments and consequences.* New York, NY: Cambridge University Press.

Cusick, A., & McCluskey, A. (2000). Becoming an evidence-based practitioner through professional development. *Australian Occupational Therapy Journal, 47*(4), 159-170.

Csikszentmihalyi, M. (1996). *Creativity: Flow and the psychology of discovery and invention.* New York, NY: HarperCollins.

Fletcher, T. (2010). A grounded theory analysis of the relationship between creativity and occupational therapy. *Dissertation Abstracts International: Section B: The Sciences and Engineering, 71*(4-B), 2324.

Furnham, A., & Bachtiar, V. (2008). Personality and intelligence as predictors of creativity. *Personality and Individual Differences, 45*(7), 613-617.

Guilford, J. P. (1950). Creativity. *American Psychologist, 5*(9), 444-454.

Guilford, J. P., & Hoepfner, R. (1971). *The analysis of intelligence.* New York, NY: McGraw-Hill.

Kalischuk, R., & Thorpe, K. (2002). Thinking creatively: From nursing education to practice. *Journal of Continuing Education in Nursing, 33*(4), 155-163.

Maslach, C., & Jackson, S. E. (1981). The measurement of experienced burnout. *Journal of Occupational Behavior, 2*(2), 99-113.

Maslow, A. (1970). *Motivation and personality* (2nd ed.). New York, NY: Harper and Row.

Mayfield, M., & Mayfield, J. (2010). Developing a scale to measure the creative environment perceptions: A questionnaire for investigating garden variety creativity. *Creativity Research Journal, 22*(2), 162-169.

Nelson, B., & Rawlings, D. (2009). How does it feel? The development of the Experience of Creativity Questionnaire. *Creativity Research Journal, 21*(1), 43-53.

O'Quin, K., and Besemer, S. P. (2006). Using the Creative Product Semantic Scale as a metric for results-oriented business. *Creativity and Innovation Management, 15*(1), 34-44.

Rodgers, C. R. (1961). *On becoming a person.* Boston, MA: Houghton Mifflin.

Roskos-Ewoldsen, B., Black, S., & McCown, S. (2008). Age-related changes in creative thinking. *Journal of Creative Behavior, 42*(1), 33-59.

Runco, M. A. (2004). Creativity. *Annual Review of Psychology, 55*(1), 657-687.

Sandovich, J. M. (2005). Work excitement in nursing: An examination of the relationship between work excitement and burnout. *Nursing Economics, 23*(2), 91-96.

Sternberg, R. (2003). *Wisdom, intelligence, and creativity synthesized.* New York, NY: Cambridge University Press.

Taylor, I. A., & Sandler, B. E. (1972). Use of a creative product inventory for evaluating products of chemists. *Proceedings of the Annual Convention of the American Psychological Association, 7*(1), 311-312.

Torrance, E. P. (1966). *Torrance Test of Creative Thinking.* Bensonville, IL: Scholastic Testing.

Torrance, E. P., & White, W. F. (1969). *Issues and advances in educational psychology.* Itasca, IL: F. E. Peacock.

Epilogue

Integrating one's life experiences with what an occupational therapy practitioner must know at entry level is challenging. As a student, developing a personal approach to treatment requires discipline as well as creativity. Role-playing what a client might feel and do with limited use of one hand or low vision to perform a task may give insight in how to work effectively with someone experiencing this difficulty and provide valuable self-knowledge. When the activity is one the student truly wants to do, then the role-play of being disabled may lead to quite a difference experience. Frustration, disappointment, or anger may result in an emotional tangle limiting creative problem solving. In an actual situation in which live clients are faced with very real problems, they look to the occupational therapy practitioner for answers. By simulating a client's situation, ideas may be generated for changing the approach or completion of the task that otherwise might not occur. In reality, a straightforward solution that the client is willing to accept may be farther away. For example, the first step may be providing a client with patient education on hip precautions, the second to discover an alternative for entering a car with bucket seats. Only opportunities to practice the activity will reveal the nuances of successful performance, the locus of control, and the amount to release or withhold for safe performance.

The therapist's behaviors and unique characteristics as an individual affect the client's response to treatment as well. Identifying one's habits, values, and roles as a student is preparation for assessing the same elements in clients to design interventions meaningful for them. The preferred learning style of the therapist may be different from the client's. Recognizing the difference exists and what to do as a result can alter a client's refusal of treatment to eager anticipation for the next session. The client's cultural background may alter one's words and phrases into the equivalent of speaking a foreign language. Identifying the effect of "slang" or speaking in layman terms can turn confusion or distrust into a desire for participating in therapy. Awareness of one's personal attributes and their effect in establishing a helping relationship takes practice and experience that starts in the classroom and continues in the clinic. Refinement of one's therapeutic use of self is a continual process congruent with choosing the environment and context to provide that "just right challenge."

The ongoing challenge for all students (and occupational therapy practitioners) is developing reasoning skills and empathetic treatment techniques coupled with flexible creativity used on a daily basis, even moment-by-moment. Professionally speaking, occupational therapy is a small world, but we treat the whole world. All the differences and similarities between students and their peers; their present experiences, past histories, and future dreams; and everything the student has ever said, felt, thought, and did (or will do) are resources, preparing them to effectively work with whoever walks through the door seeking occupational therapy treatment. That difficult or pleasant, joking or whining, demanding or submissive, mature or immature peer may be tomorrow's client. As an entry-level practitioner, how will the student respond? This is the reality they are being prepared to meet. Continual reflection on their own life will serve them well. In other words, students are involved in a life-long journey toward understanding occupation. Every moment has the potential to be an epiphany, now or in some forthcoming context, for providing occupational therapy.

Our intent in providing this textbook is to help students become practitioners who intuitively and creatively adjust their approaches and interventions to what clients need to succeed. This is the basic philosophy that occupational therapy has embraced throughout its history: "Our role consists in giving opportunities rather than prescriptions..." (Meyer, 1977, p. 7). Our expectation is that students will become those who instill trust, hope, and the rapport needed to create a working relationship to carry through meaningful intervention. As time goes by, each student will develop a distinct "flavor" and "style" of delivery in providing occupational therapy treatment. Helping clients arrive at a level of comfort and confidence in performing their occupations is therapy and enabling them to engage creatively in their occupations is the most important aspect of their lives.

REFERENCE

Meyer, A. (1977). The philosophy of occupation therapy. Reprinted from the *Archives of Occupational Therapy*, Volume 1, pp. 1-10, 1922. *American Journal of Occupational Therapy, 31*(10), 639-642.

Coffey MS, Lamport NK, Hersch GI.
Creative Engagement in Occupation: Building Professional Skills (p 109).
© 2015 SLACK Incorporated.

Appendix

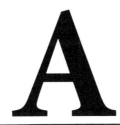

Diagrams for the Occupational Therapy Practice Framework

Six Aspects of Occupational Therapy's Domain

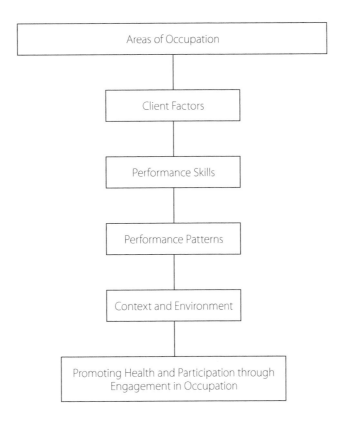

Areas of Occupation

Client Factors

Performance Skills

Performance Patterns

Context and Environment

Promoting Health and Participation through Engagement in Occupation

Appendix A is reprinted with permission from American Occupational Therapy Association. (2008). *Occupational therapy practice framework: Domain and process* (2nd ed.). Bethesda, MD: American Occupational Therapy Association.

Coffey MS, Lamport NK, Hersch GI.
Creative Engagement in Occupation: Building Professional Skills (pp 111-117).
© 2015 SLACK Incorporated.

MAJOR CATEGORIES FOR EACH OF THE
SIX OCCUPATIONAL THERAPY DOMAINS

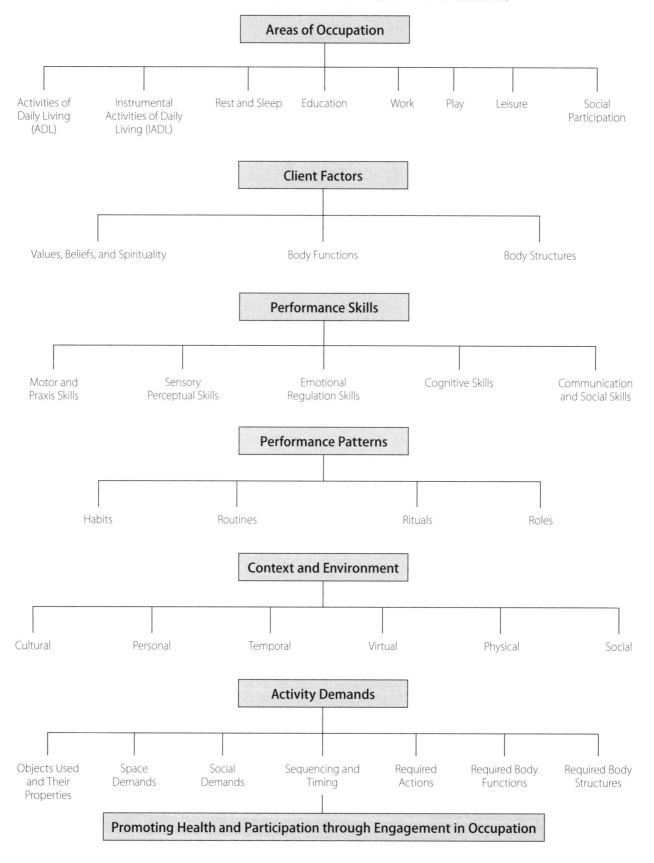

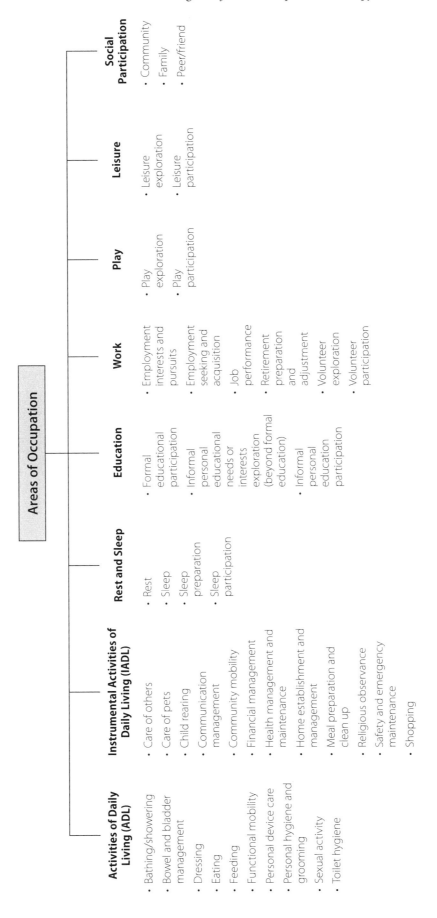

Areas of Occupation

Activities of Daily Living (ADL)
- Bathing/showering
- Bowel and bladder management
- Dressing
- Eating
- Feeding
- Functional mobility
- Personal device care
- Personal hygiene and grooming
- Sexual activity
- Toilet hygiene

Instrumental Activities of Daily Living (IADL)
- Care of others
- Care of pets
- Child rearing
- Communication management
- Community mobility
- Financial management
- Health management and maintenance
- Home establishment and management
- Meal preparation and clean up
- Religious observance
- Safety and emergency maintenance
- Shopping

Rest and Sleep
- Rest
- Sleep
- Sleep preparation
- Sleep participation

Education
- Formal educational participation
- Informal personal educational needs or interests exploration (beyond formal education)
- Informal personal education participation

Work
- Employment interests and pursuits
- Employment seeking and acquisition
- Job performance
- Retirement preparation and adjustment
- Volunteer exploration
- Volunteer participation

Play
- Play exploration
- Play participation

Leisure
- Leisure exploration
- Leisure participation

Social Participation
- Community
- Family
- Peer/friend

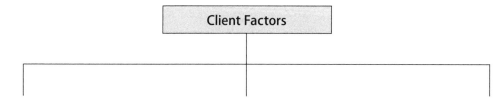

Client Factors

Values, Beliefs, and Spirituality

- Person
- Organization
- Population

Body Function Categories

- Mental functions
  - Global
  - Specific
- Sensory functions and pain
  - Seeing
  - Hearing/vestibular
  - Taste/smell/proprioceptive
  - Touch/pain/temperature/ pressure
- Neuromusculoskeletal and movement-related functions
  - Joints and bones
  - Muscle power, endurance, involuntary and voluntary movements
  - Gait patterns
- Cardiovascular, hematological, immunological, and respiratory system function
- Voice and speech functions
- Digestive, metabolic, and endocrine system
- Genitourinary and reproductive
- Skin and hair/nails

Body Structure Categories

- Nervous system
- Eye, ear
- Voice/speech
- Cardiovascular, immunological, respiratory
- Digestive, metabolic, endocrine
- Genitourinary and reproductive
- Movement
- Skin and hair/nails

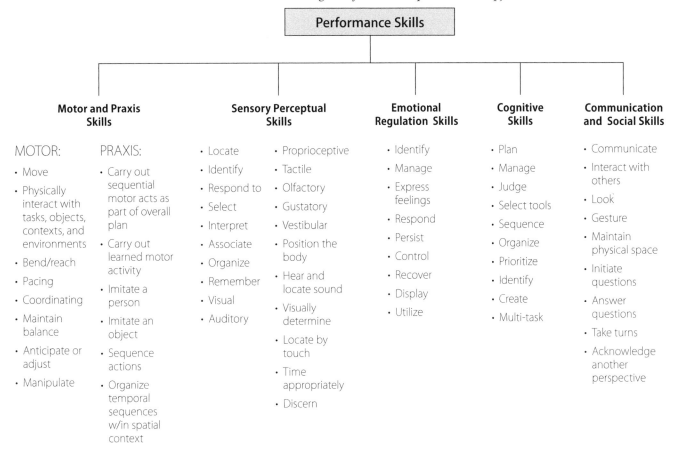

Performance Skills

Motor and Praxis Skills

MOTOR:
- Move
- Physically interact with tasks, objects, contexts, and environments
- Bend/reach
- Pacing
- Coordinating
- Maintain balance
- Anticipate or adjust
- Manipulate

PRAXIS:
- Carry out sequential motor acts as part of overall plan
- Carry out learned motor activity
- Imitate a person
- Imitate an object
- Sequence actions
- Organize temporal sequences w/in spatial context

Sensory Perceptual Skills
- Locate
- Identify
- Respond to
- Select
- Interpret
- Associate
- Organize
- Remember
- Visual
- Auditory
- Proprioceptive
- Tactile
- Olfactory
- Gustatory
- Vestibular
- Position the body
- Hear and locate sound
- Visually determine
- Locate by touch
- Time appropriately
- Discern

Emotional Regulation Skills
- Identify
- Manage
- Express feelings
- Respond
- Persist
- Control
- Recover
- Display
- Utilize

Cognitive Skills
- Plan
- Manage
- Judge
- Select tools
- Sequence
- Organize
- Prioritize
- Identify
- Create
- Multi-task

Communication and Social Skills
- Communicate
- Interact with others
- Look
- Gesture
- Maintain physical space
- Initiate questions
- Answer questions
- Take turns
- Acknowledge another perspective

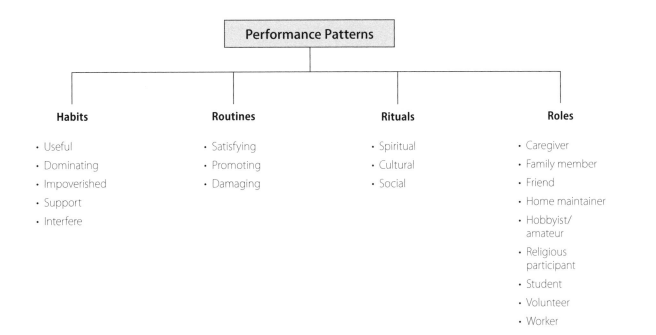

Performance Patterns

Habits
- Useful
- Dominating
- Impoverished
- Support
- Interfere

Routines
- Satisfying
- Promoting
- Damaging

Rituals
- Spiritual
- Cultural
- Social

Roles
- Caregiver
- Family member
- Friend
- Home maintainer
- Hobbyist/ amateur
- Religious participant
- Student
- Volunteer
- Worker

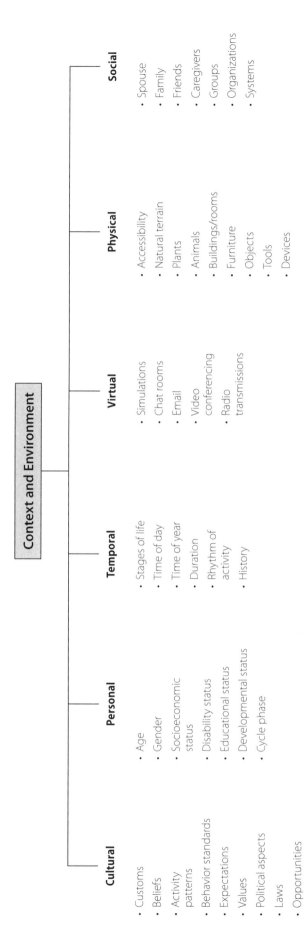

Context and Environment

Cultural
- Customs
- Beliefs
- Activity patterns
- Behavior standards
- Expectations
- Values
- Political aspects
- Laws
- Opportunities

Personal
- Age
- Gender
- Socioeconomic status
- Disability status
- Educational status
- Developmental status
- Cycle phase

Temporal
- Stages of life
- Time of day
- Time of year
- Duration
- Rhythm of activity
- History

Virtual
- Simulations
- Chat rooms
- Email
- Video conferencing
- Radio transmissions

Physical
- Accessibility
- Natural terrain
- Plants
- Animals
- Buildings/rooms
- Furniture
- Objects
- Tools
- Devices

Social
- Spouse
- Family
- Friends
- Caregivers
- Groups
- Organizations
- Systems

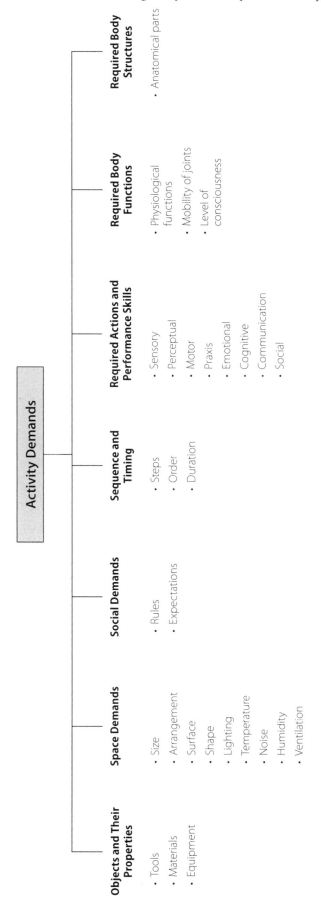

Activity Demands

Objects and Their Properties
- Tools
- Materials
- Equipment

Space Demands
- Size
- Arrangement
- Surface
- Shape
- Lighting
- Temperature
- Noise
- Humidity
- Ventilation

Social Demands
- Rules
- Expectations

Sequence and Timing
- Steps
- Order
- Duration

Required Actions and Performance Skills
- Sensory
- Perceptual
- Motor
- Praxis
- Emotional
- Cognitive
- Communication
- Social

Required Body Functions
- Physiological functions
- Mobility of joints
- Level of consciousness

Required Body Structures
- Anatomical parts

Appendix

B

Literature Review on Creativity and Occupational Therapy

Adams-Price, C. E., & Steinman, B. A. (2007). Crafts and generative expression: A qualitative study of the meaning of creativity in women who make jewelry in midlife. *International Journal of Aging and Human Development, 65*(4), 315-333.

Arbesman, M., & Puccio, G. (2001). Enhanced quality through creative problem solving. *Journal of Nursing Administration, 31*(4), 176-178.

Baycrest. (2010). Arts for life: Taking a scientific look at how creativity supports healthy aging. Retrieved from http://www.baycrest.org/Breakthroughs/Winter2010/artslife.html.

Breines, E. B. (2004). Rabbi Emil Gustave Hirsch: Ethical philosopher and founding figure of occupational therapy. In *Occupational therapy: Activities for practice and teaching.* London, UK: Whurr Publishers.

Brown, C. A. (Ed.) (2009). *Selected resources for occupational therapy practice: A review of current issues.* Alberta, Canada: University of Alberta.

Caldwell, L. L. (2005). Leisure and health: Why is leisure therapeutic? *British Journal of Guidance & Counselling, 33*(1), 7-26.

Carter, B. A., Nelson, D. L., & Duncombe, L. W. (1983). The effect of psychological type on the mood and meaning of two collage activities. *American Journal of Occupational Therapy, 37*(10), 688-693.

Casteleijn, D., & de Vos, H. (2007). The model of creative ability in vocational rehabilitation. *Work, 29*(1), 55-61.

Cipriani, J., Haley, R. Moravec, E., & Young. H. (2010). Experience and meaning of group altruistic activities among long-term care residents. *British Journal of Occupational Therapy, 73*(6), 269-276.

Cohen, G. D. (2005). *The mature mind: The positive power of the aging brain.* New York, NY: Basic Books.

Fletcher, T. (2010). A grounded theory analysis of the relationship between creativity and occupational therapy. *Dissertation Abstracts International: Section B: The Sciences and Engineering, 71*(4-B), 2324.

Fletcher, T. (2011). Creative thinking in schools: Finding the "just right" challenge for students. *Gifted Child Today, 34*(2), 37-42.

Florey, L. L. (1981). Studies of play: Implications for growth, development, and for clinical practice. *American Journal of Occupational Therapy, 35*(8), 519-524.

Frye, B. (1990). Art and multiple personality disorder: An expressive framework for occupational therapy. *American Journal of Occupational Therapy, 44*(11), 1013-1022.

Coffey MS, Lamport NK, Hersch GI.
Creative Engagement in Occupation: Building Professional Skills (pp 119-121).
© 2015 SLACK Incorporated.

Griffiths, S. (2008). The experience of creative activity as a treatment medium. *Journal of Mental Health, 17*(1), 49-63.

Griffiths, S., & Corr, S. (2007). The use of creative activities with people with mental health problems: A survey of occupational therapists. *British Journal of Occupational Therapy, 70*(3), 107-114.

Guitard, P., Ferland, F., & Dutil, E. (2005). Toward a better understanding of playfulness in adults. *OTJR: Occupation, Participation and Health, 25*(1), 9-22. Retrieved from http://otj.sagepub.com/content/25/1/9.full.pdf+html .

Hasselkus, B. R., & Murray, B. J. (2007). Everyday occupation, well-being, and identity: The experience of caregivers in families with dementia. *American Journal of Occupational Therapy, 61*(1), 9-20.

Henare, D., Hocking, C., & Smythe. L. (2003). Chronic pain: Gaining understanding through the use of art. *British Journal of Occupational Therapy, 66*(1), 511-518.

Hinojosa, J. (2007). Becoming innovators in the era of hyperchange. *American Journal of Occupational Therapy, 61*(6), 629-637.

Howie, L., Coulter, M., & Feldman, S. (2004). Crafting the self: Older persons' narratives of occupational identity. *American Journal of Occupational Therapy, 58*(4), 446-454.

Josephsson, S., Asaba, E., Jonsson, H., & Alsaker, S. (2006). Creativity and order in communication: Implications from philosophy to narrative research concerning human occupation. *Scandinavian Journal of Occupational Therapy, 13*(2), 86-93.

King L. J. (1980). Creative caring. *American Journal of Occupational Therapy, 34*(8), 522-528.

La Cour, K., Josephsson, S., & Luborsky, M. (2005). Creating connections to life during life-threatening illness: Creative activity experienced by elderly people and occupational therapists. *Scandinavian Journal of Occupational Therapy, 12*(3), 98-109.

Lederer, J. M. (2007). Disposition toward critical thinking among occupational therapy students. *American Journal of Occupational Therapy, 61*(5), 519-526.

Lehrer, J. (2010, February 19). Peak performance: Fleeting youth and fading creativity. *Wall Street Journal.* Retrieved from http://online.wsj.com/news/articles/SB40001424052748703444804575071573334216604.

Levine, R. (1987). Looking back: The influence of the arts-and-crafts movement on the professional status of occupational therapy. *American Journal of Occupational Therapy, 41*(4), 248-254.

Murray, C. (2010). Fostering student creativity. *OT Practice, 15*(17), 9-12.

Nilsson, I., Bernspång, B., Fisher, A. G., Gustafson, Y., & Löfgren, B. (2007). Occupational engagement and life satisfaction in the oldest-old: The Umeå 85+ study. *OTJR: Occupation, Participation and Health, 27*(4), 131-139. Retrieved from http://www.slackjournals.com/article.aspx?rid=24556.

Oliviero, H. (2011, June 8). Garden therapy helpful to patients. *The Atlanta Journal-Constitution.* Retrieved from http://www.ajc.com/news/lifestyles/garden-therapy-helpful-to-patients/nQt7g/.

Peloquin, S. (1996). Art: An occupation with promise for developing empathy. *American Journal of Occupational Therapy, 50*(8), 655-661.

Peloquin, S. (1994). Occupational therapy as art and science: Should the older definition be reclaimed? *American Journal of Occupational Therapy, 48*(11), 1093-1094.

Peloquin, S. (1996). Brief or new: Using the arts to enhance confluent learning. *American Journal of Occupational Therapy, 50*(2), 148-151.

Peloquin, S. (2006). Occupations: Strands of coherence in a life. *American Journal of Occupational Therapy, 60*(2), 236-239.

Perruzza, N., & Kinsella, E. A. (2010). Creative arts occupations in therapeutic practice: A review of the literature. *British Journal of Occupational Therapy, 73*(6), 261-268.

Price, P., & Cashman, J. (1996). Jenny's story: Reinventing oneself through occupation and narrative configuration. *American Journal of Occupational Therapy, 50*(4), 306-314.

Price, P., & Miner, S. (2007) Occupation emerges in the process of therapy. *American Journal of Occupational Therapy, 61*(4), 441-450.

Reynolds, F. (2009). Taking up arts and crafts in later life: A qualitative study of the experiential factors that encourage participation in creative activities. *British Journal of Occupational Therapy, 72*(9), 393-400.

Reynolds, F. (2009). Creative occupations: A need for in-depth longitudinal qualitative studies. *British Journal of Occupational Therapy, 72*(1), 1.

Reynolds, F., Vivat, B., & Prior, S. (2008). Women's experiences of increasing subjective well-being in CFS/ME through leisure-based arts and crafts activities: A qualitative study. *Disability and Rehabilitation, 30*(17), 1279-1288.

Robinson, K., Kennedy, N., & Harmon, D. (2011). Is occupational therapy adequately meeting the needs of people with chronic pain? *American Journal of Occupational Therapy, 65*(1), 106-113.

Sudhakar, G., & Le Blanc, M. (2011). Alternate splint for flexion contracture in children with burns. *Journal of Hand Therapy, 24*(3), 277-279.

Symons, J., Clark, H., Williams, K., Hansen, E., & Orpin, P. (2011). Visual art in physical rehabilitation: Experiences of people with neurological conditions. *British Journal of Occupational Therapy, 74*(1), 44-52.

Taylor, L. P. S., & McGruder, J. E. (1996). The meaning of sea kayaking for persons with spinal cord injuries. *American Journal of Occupational Therapy, 50*(1), 39-46.

Wallenbert, I., & Jonsson, H. (2005). Waiting to get better: A dilemma regarding habits in daily occupations after stroke. *American Journal of Occupational Therapy, 59*(2), 218-224.

Weinstein, E. (1998). Elements of the art of practice in mental health. *American Journal of Occupational Therapy, 52*(7), 579-585.

Williams, S., & Paterson, M. (2009). A phenomenological study of the art of occupational therapy. *The Qualitative Report, 14*(4), 689-718. Retrieved from http://www.nova.edu/ssss/QR/QR14-4/williams.pdf.

Wood, W. (2007). Associate editor's note: The sustaining power of ideas. *American Journal of Occupational Therapy, 61*(5), 597-598. Retrieved from http://ajot.aota.org/article.aspx?articleid=1866995.

Wright, J., Sadlo, G., & Stew, G. (2006). Challenge-skills and mindfulness: An exploration of the conundrum of flow process. *OTJR: Occupation, Participation and Health, 26*(1), 25-32. Retrieved from http://www.slackjournals.com/article.aspx?rid=5099.

Appendix

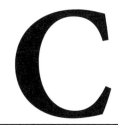

Table of
Quantitative Assessment Methods

Tina Fletcher, EdD, MFA, OTR

TEST NAME/ AUTHOR(S)	SOURCE	COST/SCORING/ ADMINISTRATION TIME	CONSTRUCTS MEASURED
Creativity			
Abbreviated Torrance Test for Adults (Kathy Goff & E. Paul Torrance, 2002)	Scholastic Testing Service, Inc., 480 Myer Rd., Bensenville, IL 60106-1617. (800) 642-6787; stesting@email.com; www.ststesting.com	$15.45 per sample kit/group administration/9 min	Designed to be a measure of creative thinking ability in people over 18 years; fluency, originality, elaboration, and flexibility, with creativity indicators
Adjective Checklist (Harrison G. Gough & Alfred B. Heilbrun, Jr., 1952-1980)	Consulting Psychologists Press, Inc., 3803 East Bayshore Rd., P.O. Box 10096, Palo Alto, CA 94303. (800) 624-1765	$8.00 per 25 checklists/group administration/15 to 20 min	Designed to identify personal characteristics of individuals; number of adjectives checked, number of favorable or unfavorable adjectives, etc.

(continued)

Coffey MS, Lamport NK, Hersch GI.
Creative Engagement in Occupation: Building Professional Skills (pp 123-129).
© 2015 SLACK Incorporated.

TEST NAME/ AUTHOR(S)	SOURCE	COST/SCORING/ ADMINISTRATION TIME	CONSTRUCTS MEASURED
Creatrix Inventory (Revised) (Richard Byrd & Jacqueline Byrd, 1971-2006)	Creatrix, 135 Black Oaks Lane, Wayzata, MN 55391. (952) 925-1751; team@creatrix.com; www.creatrix.com	$5.95 per manual/ group administration, online administration and scoring/ no time report	Designed for self-assessment and educational purposes; determines a person's creative risk-taking propensity; creativity, risk taking, sustainer, modifier, challenger, practicalizer, innovator, synthesizer, dreamer, planner
KEYS to Creativity (Teresa Amabile, 1995)	Center for Creative Leadership, One Leadership Place, P.O. Box 26300, Greensboro, NC 27438-6300. (336) 288-7210; info@leaders. ccl.org; www.ccl.org	$20 per survey booklet/group administration/15 to 20 min	Designed to measure how employees perceive stimulants and barriers to creativity; organizational encouragement of creativity, supervisory encouragement of creativity, work group supports, freedom, sufficient resources, challenging work, organizational impediments, workload pressure, creativity, productivity
Khatena-Torrance Creative Perception Inventory (E. Paul Torrance & Joe Khatena, 1976-1998)	Scholastic Testing Service, Inc., 480 Myer Rd., Bensenville, IL 60106-1617. (800) 642-6787; stesting@email. com; www.ststesting. com	$57.65 per starter kit/ group administration/10 to 20 min per checklist (two total)	Developed as measures of creative personality; acceptance of authority, self-confidence, inquisitiveness, awareness of others, disciplined imagination, environmental sensitivity, initiative, self-strength, intellectuality, individuality, artistry
Kirton Adaption-Innovation Inventory (Michael Kirton, 1976-1998)	Occupational Research Centre, "Cornerways" Cardigan St., Newmarket, Suffolk CBB 8HZ, United Kingdom. j.kirton@kaicentre.com; www.kaicentre.com	No price data/ individual or group administration/5 to 10 min	A measure of a person's preference for or style of creativity, problem solving, and decision making; sufficiency vs proliferation of originality, efficiency, rule/ group conformity, etc.; must be certified
Quality of Life Inventory (Michael Frisch, 1994)	NCS, 5605 Green Circle Dr., Minnetonka, MN 55343	$80.00 per starter kit/individual or group administration/5 min	Developed to provide a measure of a person's quality of life and their satisfaction with life; 17 factors (health, self-esteem, goals and values, money, work, play, learning, creativity, helping, love, friends, children, relatives, home, neighborhood, community, overall quality of life)

(continued)

TEST NAME/ AUTHOR(S)	SOURCE	COST/SCORING/ ADMINISTRATION TIME	CONSTRUCTS MEASURED
Sixteen Personality Factor Questionnaire (Raymond Cattell, Karen Cattell, Heather Cattell, Darcie Karol, & Mary Russell, 1949-1994)	Institute for Personality and Ability Testing, Inc., P.O. Box 1188, Champaign, IL 61824-1188	$82.00 per kit/group administration, computer scoring option/25 to 50 min	Designed to measure personality traits, 16 primary factor scores, five global factor scores (extraverted vs introverted, high vs low anxiety, tough-minded vs receptive, independent vs accommodating, self-controlled vs unrestrained), and three response style indices (impression management, infrequency, acquiescence)
Torrance Tests of Creative Thinking (E. Paul Torrance, 1966-1984)	Scholastic Testing Service, Inc., 480 Myer Rd., Bensenville, IL 60106-1617. (800) 642-6787. stesting@email.com; www.ststesting.com	$28.95 per 20/individual or group administration/30 to 45 min	To identify and evaluate creative potential, verbal, figural, fluency, flexibility, originality, elaboration
Trait Evaluation Index (Nelson Alan, 1967-1984)	Martin M. Bruce, Ph.D., 22516 Caravelle Circle, Boca Raton, FL 33433-5909; (561) 393-2428; brucepubl@adelphia.net	$94.20 per test package/group administration/30 to 50 min	Designed to elicit comprehensive, multidimensional appraisals of normal personality dimensions; social orientation, compliance, benevolence, elation, ambition, motivational drive, self-confidence, dynamism, independence, personal adequacy, caution, self-organization, responsibility, propriety, courtesy, verbal orientation, intellectual orientation, perception, self-control, fair-mindedness, adaptability, sincerity, overall adjustment, masculinity, femininity, consistency, employment stability, productivity, creativity, job satisfaction
Personality			
Coopersmith Self-Esteem Inventories (Stanley Coopersmith, 1981)	Consulting Psychologists Press, Inc., 3803 East Bayshore Rd., P.O. Box 10096, Palo Alto, CA 94303	$7.50 per manual/group administration/10 to 15 min	Designed to measure evaluative attitudes toward the self in social, academic, family, and personal areas of experience; general self, social self–peers, home–parents, school–academic, total self-score

(continued)

TEST NAME/ AUTHOR(S)	SOURCE	COST/SCORING/ ADMINISTRATION TIME	CONSTRUCTS MEASURED
Five Factor Wellness Inventory (Jane Myers & Thomas Sweeney, 2005)	Mind Garden, Inc., 855 Oak Grove Ave., Suite 215, Menlo Park, CA 94025	$40 per manual, $10 web administration per report, $160 for 20 of one version/ group administration/10 to 20 min	Designed to assess characters of wellness as a basis for helping individuals make choices for healthier living, wellness creative self, coping self, social self, essential self, physical self, local context, institutional context, global context, chronometrical context, life satisfaction index
Gordon Personal Profile– Inventory (Revised) (Leonard Gordon, 1951-1993)	The Psychological Corporation, 555 Academic Court, San Antonio, TX 78204-2498	$45 per complete kit/group administration/20 to 25 min	Constructed to assess eight important factors in the personality domain; ascendancy, responsibility, emotional stability, sociability, self-esteem (total), Gordon Personal Inventory, four scores (cautiousness, original thinking, personal relations, vigor)
Millon Index of Personality Styles (Revised) (Theodore Millon, 1994-2004)	Pearson, 5601 Green Valley Dr., Bloomington, MN 55437	$169.00 per starter kit/individual or group administration/25 to 30 min	Designed to measure personality styles of normally functioning adults; six motivating styles, eight thinking styles, 10 behavior styles, three validity indices, clinical index
NEO-4 (Paul Costa & Robert McCrae, 1998)	Psychological Assessment Resources, Inc., P.O. Box 998, Odessa, FL 33556	$219.00/individual or group administration/25 to 35 min	Designed as a four-factor version of the Revised NEO Personality Inventory (extraversion, openness to experience, agreeableness, conscientiousness)
NEO-FF (Paul Costa & Robert McCrae, 1978-1992)	Psychological Assessment Resources, Inc., P.O. Box 998, Odessa, FL 33556	$71.00/individual or group administration/10 to 15 min	Designed to measure five major dimensions or domains of normal adult personality; 60-item short version of NEO-PI-R; offers domain scores (neuroticism, extraversion, openness, agreeableness, conscientiousness) but no facets
NEO-PI-R (Paul Costa & Robert McCrae, 1978-1992)	Psychological Assessment Resources, Inc., P.O. Box 998, Odessa, FL 33556	$92.00/individual or group administration/30 to 40 min	Designed to measure the five major dimensions or domains of normal adult personality; 35 scores (30 facets in five domains: neuroticism, extraversion, openness, agreeableness, conscientiousness)

(continued)

TEST NAME/ AUTHOR(S)	SOURCE	COST/SCORING/ ADMINISTRATION TIME	CONSTRUCTS MEASURED
Six Factor Personality Questionnaire (Douglas Jackson, Sampo Paunonen, & Paul Tremblay, 1967-2000)	Sigma Assessment Systems, 511 Fort St., Suite 435, Port Huron, MI 48061. Robin, extension 229; www.sigmaassessmentsystems.com	75.00 per kit plus 40% research discount/computer or machine score, individual or group administration/ 20 min	Designed as a measure of six personality dimensions or broad factors (extraversion, agreeableness, independence, openness to experience, methodicalness, industriousness)
Work/Vocational			
Maslach Burnout Inventory (3rd ed.) (Christina Maslach, Susan Jackson, Michael Leiter, & Wilmar Schaufeli, 1981-1996)	CPP, Inc., 3803 East Bayshore Rd., Palo Alto, CA 94303	$65.00 review book/ group administration/5 to 15 min	Constructed to measure three aspects of burnout (emotional exhaustion, depersonalization, personal accomplishment)
Meeker Behavioral Correlates (Mary Meeker, 1981)	SOI Systems, 45755 Goodpasture Rd., P.O. Box D, Vida, OR 97488	No price data/group administration/ 20 min	Assesses major dimensions of intellectual abilities and personality for management matching of teams Comprehension, memory, leadership, convergent production skills, creativity, team contributions
Meta-Motivation Inventory (John Walker, 1979)	Meta-Visions, 5076 Queen Victoria Lane, Kalamazoo, MI 49009-7799. (616) 353-9577; jwalker@aol.com	No price data/group administration/no time data	Self-administered, managers and persons in leadership positions; motivation for achievement, perfection, assertiveness, independence, achievement, meta-achievement, deterministic, approval, conventional, dependent, avoidance, helplessness, need for control, persuasiveness, manipulation, reactive, authoritarian, exploitive, concern for people, cooperation, affiliation, humanistic, synergy, meta-humanistic, self-actualization, stress, repression, anger, judgmental, creativity, growth potential, fun scales

(continued)

TEST NAME/ AUTHOR(S)	SOURCE	COST/SCORING/ ADMINISTRATION TIME	CONSTRUCTS MEASURED
Minnesota Importance Questionnaire (James Rounds, Jr., George Henley, René Dawis, Lloyd Lofquist, & David Weiss, 1967-1981)	Vocational Psychology Research, N6112 Elliott Hall, University of Minnesota-Twin Cities, 75 East River Rd., Minneapolis, MN 55455-0344. (612) 625-1367. vpr@tc.umn.edu; www.psych.umn.edu/psylabs/vpr	2001: $39.50 complete kit/group administration, scoring service option/15 to 25 min (ranked form) and 30 to 40 min (paired form)	To measure 20 psychological needs and six underlying values found to be relevant to work adjustment, specifically to satisfaction with work; ability utilization, achievement activity, independence variety compensation, security, working conditions, advancement, recognition, authority, social status, coworkers, social services, moral values, company policies, supervision-human relations, supervision-technical, creativity, responsibility, autonomy
Minnesota Job Description Questionnaire (Fred Borgen, David Weiss, Howard Tinsley, René Dawis, & Lloyd Lofquist, 1967-1968)	Vocational Psychology Research, N6112 Elliott Hall, University of Minnesota-Twin Cities, 75 East River Rd., Minneapolis, MN 55455-0344. (612) 625-1367. vpr@tc.umn.edu; www.psych.umn.edu/psylabs/vpr	2001: $0.73 per copy/group administration, scoring service option/20 min	Designed to measure the reinforced characteristics of jobs; ability utilization, achievement, activity, advancement, authority, company policies and practices, compensation, coworkers, creativity, independence, moral values, recognition, responsibility, security, social service, social status, supervision-human relations, supervision-technical, variety, working conditions, autonomy
Minnesota Multi-phasic Personality Inventory-2 (Starke Hathaway, J. C. McKinley, & James Butcher, 1942-1990)	University of Minnesota Press, National Computer Systems, Inc., Professional Assessment Services Division, P.O. Box 1416, Minneapolis, MN 55440	1989: $17.70 per 10 reusable books/group administration/90 min	Designed to assess a number of the major patterns of personality and emotional disorders; validity factors, 15 supplementary scales, 15 content scales, three SI subscales, 28 Harris-Lingoes subscales
Staff Burnout Scale for Health Professionals (John Jones, 1980)	SRA/London House, 9701 West Higgins Rd., Rosemead, IL 60018	1992: $20.00 per 35 booklets/individual or group administration/10 min	To assess burnout or work stress
Supers Work Values Inventory (Donald Super & Donald Zytowski, 2001)	National Career Assessment Services, Inc., 302 Visions Parkway, Adel, IA 50003-1632. (800) 314-8972; ncasi@ncasi.com, www.kuder.com	No price data/individual or group administration, online and instant scoring/15 to 20 min	Assesses relative importance of selected attributes of occupation and jobs; achievement, coworkers, creativity, income, independence, lifestyle mental challenge, prestige, security, supervision, work environment, variety

(continued)

TEST NAME/ AUTHOR(S)	SOURCE	COST/SCORING/ ADMINISTRATION TIME	CONSTRUCTS MEASURED
Work Personality Index (Donald Macnab & Shawn Bakker, 2001)	Psychometrics Canada Ltd., 7125-77 Ave., Edmonton, Alberta, T6B 0B5, Canada	No price data/ individual or group administration, paper and pencil or internet scoring/20 to 40 min	Designed to identify personality traits that directly relate to work performance (teamwork, concern for others, outgoing, democratic, attention to detail, rule-following, dependability, ambition energy, persistence, leadership, innovation, analytic thinking, self-control, stress, tolerance, initiative, flexibility, achievement, conscientiousness, social orientation, practical intelligence, adjustment)

Appendix

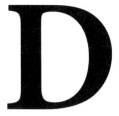

Suggested Resources
Creativity and Occupational Therapy

AMERICAN JOURNAL OF OCCUPATIONAL THERAPY ARTICLES

Friedland, J. (2009). Evolving identities: Thomas Bessell Kidner and occupational therapy in the United States. *American Journal of Occupational Therapy, 62*(3), 349-360.

Gillette, N. (2008). A firm persuasion in our work: Mentors I have known (and loved). *American Journal of Occupational Therapy, 62*(4), 487-490.

Haak, M., Fänge, A., Horstmann, V., & Iwarsson, S. (2008). Two dimensions of participation in very old age and their relations to home and neighborhood environments. *American Journal of Occupational Therapy, 62*(1), 77-86.

Hasselkus, B. R., & Murray, B. J. (2007). Everyday occupations, well-being, and identity: The experience of caregivers in families with dementia. *American Journal of Occupational Therapy, 61*(1), 9-20.

Hinojosa, J. (2007). Becoming innovators in the era of hyperchange. *American Journal of Occupational Therapy, 61*(6), 629-637.

Hooper, B. (2008). Stories we teach by: Intersections among faculty biography, student formation, and instructional processes. *American Journal of Occupational Therapy, 62*(2), 228-241.

Howie, L., Coulter, M., & Feldman, S. (2004). Crafting the self: Older persons' narratives of occupational identity. *American Journal of Occupational Therapy, 58*(4), 446-454.

Law, M. C. (2007). A firm persuasion in our work: Occupational therapy: A journey driven by curiosity. *American Journal of Occupational Therapy, 61*(5), 599-602.

Lederer, J. M. (2007). Disposition toward critical thinking among occupational therapy students. *American Journal of Occupational Therapy, 61*(5), 519-526.

Miner, S., & Price, P. (2007). Occupation emerges in the process of therapy. *American Journal of Occupational Therapy, 61*(4), 441-450.

Peloquin, S. M. (2006). Occupations: Strands of coherence in a life. *American Journal of Occupational Therapy, 60*(2), 236-239.

Coffey MS, Lamport NK, Hersch GI.
Creative Engagement in Occupation: Building Professional Skills (pp 131-132).
© 2015 SLACK Incorporated.

Taylor, R. R., Lee, S. W., Kielhofner, G., & Ketkar, M. (2009). Therapeutic use of self: A nationwide survey of practitioners' attitudes and experiences. *American Journal of Occupational Therapy, 63*(2), 198-207.

Wallenbert, I., & Jonsson, H. (2005). Waiting to get better: A dilemma regarding habits in daily occupations after stroke. *American Journal of Occupational Therapy, 59*(2), 218-224.

Wood, W., Womack, J., & Hooper, B. (2009). Dying of boredom: An exploratory case study of time use, apparent affect and routine activity situation on two Alzheimer's special care units. *American Journal of Occupational Therapy, 63*(3), 337-350.

Yuen, H. K., Huang, P., Burik, J. K., & Smith, T. G. (2008). Impact of participating in volunteer activities for residents living in LTC facilities. *American Journal of Occupational Therapy, 62*(1), 71-76.

Zimolag, U., & Krupa, T. (2009). Pet ownership as a meaningful community occupation for people with serious mental illness. *American Journal of Occupational Therapy, 63*(2), 126-137.

OTJR: Occupation, Participation and Health Articles

Guitard, P., Ferland, F. & Dutil, E. (2005). Toward a better understanding of playfulness in adults. *OTJR: Occupation, Participation and Health, 25*(1), 9-22.

Martin, L. M., Bliven, M., & Boisvert, R. (2008). Occupational performance, self-esteem and quality of life in substance addictions recovery. *OTJR: Occupation, Participation and Health, 28*(2), 81-88.

Nilsson, I., Fisher, A. G., & Gustafson, Y. (2007). Occupational engagement and life satisfaction in the oldest-old: The Umea 85+ study. *OTJR: Occupation, Participation and Health, 27*(4), 131-139.

White, J. H., Mackenzie, L., Magin, P., & Pollack, M. R. P. (2008). The occupational experience of stroke survivors in a community setting. *OTJR: Occupation, Participation and Health, 28*(4), 160-167.

Wright, J. J., Sadlo, G., & Stew, G. (2006). Challenge-skills and mindfulness: An exploration of the conundrum of flow process. *OTJR: Occupation, Participation and Health, 26*(1), 25-32.

OT Practice Articles

Reed, K. L. (2006). Values and beliefs: The formative years: 1904-1929. *OT Practice, 11*(7), 21-25.

Reed, K. L., & Peters, C. (2006) Values and beliefs, part II: The Great Depression and war years: 1930-1949. *OT Practice, 11*(18), 17-22.

Book

Kronenberg, F., Algado, S. S., & Pollard, N. (Eds.) (2001). *Occupational therapy without borders: Learning from the spirit of survivors.* New York, NY: Elsevier.

Financial Disclosures

Dr. Mary Frances Baxter has no financial or proprietary interest in the materials presented herein.

Margaret S. Coffey has no financial or proprietary interest in the materials presented herein.

Harriett A. Davidson has no financial or proprietary interest in the materials presented herein.

Dr. Tina Fletcher has no financial or proprietary interest in the materials presented herein.

Dr. Gayle I. Hersch has no financial or proprietary interest in the materials presented herein.

Nancy K. Lamport has no financial or proprietary interest in the materials presented herein.

Dr. Marsha Neville has no financial or proprietary interest in the materials presented herein.

Index